**Third Edit**

# Clinical Methods in
# Psychiatry

# Third Edition
# Clinical Methods in
# Psychiatry

## VMD Namboodiri
BSc, MBBS, MA (Psy), MD (Psych)

Consultant Psychiatrist and Medical Director
Sevana Hospital, Pattambi Kerala

ex-Senior Consultant and Head,
Department of Psychiatry, and Joint Director
Malankara Orthodox Syrian Church Medical Mission
Medical College and Hospital, Kolenchery Kerala

## CJ John
MBBS, DPM, MD (NIMHANS), MNAMS (Psy)

Consultant Psychiatrist
Medical Trust Hospital, Ernakulam

## TP Subhalakshmi
MBBS, DPM, MD (CMC Vellore)

Consultant Psychiatrist
Malankara Orthodox Syrian Church Medical Mission
Medical College and Hospital
Kolenchery

## CBS
# CBS Publishers & Distributors Pvt Ltd

New Delhi • Bengaluru • Chennai • Kochi • Kolkata • Mumbai
Hyderabad • Nagpur • Patna • Pune • Vijayawada

Third Edition
## Clinical Methods in Psychiatry

**ISBN:** 978-81-239-2955-2

Copyright © Editors and Publisher

**Third Edition:** 2016

Second Edition: 1999

First Edition: 1984

Published by Satish Kumar Jain and produced by Varun Jain for
**CBS Publishers & Distributors** Pvt Ltd
4819/XI Prahlad Street, 24 Ansari Road, Daryaganj, New Delhi 110 002, India.
Ph: 23289259, 23266861, 23266867    Website: www.cbspd.com
Fax: 011-23243014    e-mail: delhi@cbspd.com; cbspubs@airtelmail.in.

*Corporate Office:* 204 FIE, Industrial Area, Patparganj, Delhi 110 092
Ph: 4934 4934    Fax: 4934 4935    e-mail: publishing@cbspd.com; publicity@cbspd.com

*Branches*

- **Bengaluru:** Seema House 2975, 17th Cross, K.R. Road,
  Banasankari 2nd Stage, Bengaluru 560 070, Karnataka
  Ph: +91-80-26771678/79    Fax: +91-80-26771680    e-mail: bangalore@cbspd.com
- **Chennai:** 7, Subbaraya Street, Shenoy Nagar, Chennai 600 030, Tamil Nadu
  Ph: +91-44-26680620, 26681266    Fax: +91-44-42032115    e-mail: chennai@cbspd.com
- **Kochi:** Ashana House, No. 39/1904, AM Thomas Road, Valanjambalam,
  Ernakulam 682 018, Kochi, Kerala
  Ph: +91-484-4059061-62-64-65    Fax: +91-484-4059065    e-mail: kochi@cbspd.com
- **Kolkata:** 6/B, Ground Floor, Rameswar Shaw Road, Kolkata-700 014, West Bengal
  Ph: +91-33-22891126, 22891127, 22891128    e-mail: kolkata@cbspd.com
- **Mumbai:** 83-C, Dr E Moses Road, Worli, Mumbai-400018, Maharashtra
  Ph: +91-22-24902340/41    Fax: +91-22-24902342    e-mail: mumbai@cbspd.com

*Representatives*

- **Hyderabad**  0-9885175004   • **Nagpur**  0-9021734563   • **Patna**  0-9334159340
- **Pune**  0-9623451994   • **Vijayawada**  0-9000660880

*Printed at India Binding House, Noida*

# Contributors

**Anju Kuruvilla** MD
Professor and Head
Department of Psychiatry
Christian Medical College, Vellore

**Bangalore N Gangadhar** MD
Professor
Department of Psychiatry
NIMHANS, Bangalore

**CJ John** MBBS, DPM, MD (NIMHANS),
MNAMS (Psy)
Consultant Psychiatrist
Medical Trust Hospital, Ernakulam

**Dharitri Ramaprasad**
MA (Psychology), DM and SP (NIMHANS),
PhD (Psychology)
Professor
RF College for Psychosocial Rehabilitation
Bangalore

**George Isaac** MBBS, FRCP (Canada),
Diplomate in Psychiatry and Child
Psychiatry of the American Board of
Psychiatry and Neurology
Consultant Psychiatrist
New York City, USA

**James T Antony** MD,
MRC Psych (Lon), DPM
Consultant Psychiatrist
Thrissoor; Professor Emeritus
Jubilee Mission Medical College and
Hospital, Thrissoor
Formerly Director and Professor of
Psychiatry and Principal
Medical College, Kozhikode

**Jyothsna Chandur**
MA (Psychology), M Phil
Clinical Psychology (NIMHANS)
Lecturer
RF College for Psychosocial
Rehabilitation, Bangalore

**K Kuruvilla** MD, FRC (Psych)
Professor Emeritus
Department of Psychiatry, PSG
Institute of Medical Sciences and
Research, Coimbatore, Formerly
Professor and Head, Department of
Psychiatry, Christian Medical College,
Vellore and PSG Institute of Medical
Sciences and Research,
Coimbatore

**KP Abdul Salam** MA, M Phil,
PhD (NIMHANS)
Consultant Clinical Psychologist
Sevana Hospital, Pattambi

**Naren P Rao** MD
Associate Professor
Department of Psychiatry
NIMHANS, Bangalore

**PM Vasudevan** MD, DPM
Consultant Psychiatrist
Govt Mental Hospital, Kozhikode

**Rajat Ray** MD
Professor and Head of the Department
of Psychiatry
Himalayan Institute of Medical
Sciences, Dehradun

**Ravi Gupta** MD
Associate Professor in Psychiatry
Himalayan Institute of Medical
Sciences, Dehradun

**R Johnson Pradeep** MD (Psychiatry)
Assistant Professor
Psychiatry, Ethics, Institutional Ethics
Committee (ICE), Human Research
Protection Programme and Community
Mental Health Programme, St John's
Medical College and Hospital, Bangalore

**Sadanand Rajkumar** MD (AIIMS)
VMO Psychiatrist and Professor
Intermediate Stay Mental Health Unit;
Professor, SMPH University of
Newcastle, New South Wales, Australia

**Sitalakshmi George** MBBS,
DPM (Vellore), MD (NIMHANS)
Consultant Psychiatrist, Ernakulam
Loudes Hospital, Renai Medicity, and
Lisie Hospital

**S Kalyanasundaram** MD
(Psychiatry)
Consultant Psychiatrist
Hon. CEO Richmond Fellowship
Society, Bangalore Branch; Principal
RF PG College for PSR, Bangalore

**S Santhakumar** MBBS, FRCP (G), MRC
Psych (Lon), DPM
Consultant Psychiatrist
Kozhikode; Formerly Ex-officio
Director, Institute of Mental Health
and Neuro Sciences, Kozhikode;
Professor of Psychiatry, Medical
College, and Advisor on Mental
Health to Govt of Kerala

**TP Subhalakshmi** MBBS, DPM,
MD (CMC Vellore)
Consultant Psychiatrist
Malankara Orthodox Syrian Church
Medical Mission
Medical College and Hospital,
Kolenchery

**VMD Namboodiri** BSc, MBBS,
MA (Psy), MD (Psych)
Consultant Psychiatrist and Medical
Director, Sevana Hospital, Pattambi
Formerly Senior Consultant, Head of
the Department of Psychiatry, and
Joint Director, Malankara Orthodox
Syrian Church Medical Mission
Medical College and Hospital,
Kolenchery

# Preface to the Third Edition

The first edition of this book was published in 1984 in connection with the Decennial Celebrations of the Psychiatry Department, Malankara Orthodox Syrian Church Medical Mission Hospital, Kolenchery, Kerala (now MOSC Medical College and Hospital) where all the editors have worked. The title of the book was *A Guide to Clinical Psychiatry*. The second edition came out in 1999 on the eve of the 25th anniversary of the Department as part of the silver jubilee celebrations. The book was published by B I Churchill Livingstone Pvt Ltd., New Delhi, and the name of the book was changed to *Clinical Methods in Psychiatry*.

The main changes in the present edition compared to the earlier editions are as follows.

1. Chapter "Introduction to Clinical Psychiatry" is omitted as the subject matter covered in that chapter is now shared in the other chapters.

2. Two chapters in the second edition, "Physical Investigations in Psychiatry" and "Psychological Assessment in Psychiatry" are now combined into a single chapter "Psychological Assessment in the Clinic".

3. Because of the above changes the present edition has only 16 chapters instead of 18 in the previous one.

4. There is change in authorship of some chapters (Chapters 4, 8, 9, and 14) because of the inconvenience of the previous authors to revise the respective chapters.

The editors thank all the contributors for their excellent work, goodwill and help in bringing out the current edition. Most of the authors are teachers with affiliation to reputed medical colleges and institutes. The editors highly value their clinical and teaching experiences—this being the main reason in inviting them to contribute chapters related to their fields of work.

The editors thank CBS Publishers & Distributors for kindly agreeing to bring out the present edition and Mr Y N Arjuna in particular, who encouraged us in our mission from the beginning till its end.

We sincerely hope that the book will be useful to the medical students and practitioners of psychiatry. We welcome suggestions for improvement which we hope to carry out in the successive editions.

**VMD Namboodiri**
**C J John**
**T P Subhalakshmi**

# Contents

    S KALAYANASUNDARAM, R JOHNSON PRADEEP

12. Examination of Stuporous and                           203
    Uncooperative Patients
    S RAJKUMAR

13. Patients Posing Special Problems                       211
    JAMES T ANTONY

14. Child and Adolescent Psychiatry                        221
    SITALAKSHMI GEORGE

15. Influence of Culture on the Phenomenology              235
    in Psychiatry
    S SANTHAKUMAR, PM VASUDEVAN

16. Psychological Assessments in the Clinic                245
    K P ABDUL SALAM

    *Appendix*                                             *253*

    *Index*                                                *261*

# 1

# The Psychiatric Interview

VMD Namboodiri

The purpose of the psychiatric interview is the first and foremost to discover the psychopathology hiding behind the facade of the presenting symptoms. During this process the origin and evolution of the patient's symptoms are studied against the background of his individuality. The examiner comes to know about the various psycho-biosocial factors which influenced the origin and progress of the disease. He also understands how the patient coped up with his symptoms all along and the strengths and weaknesses of his personality. The interview also demarcates the areas where further probing and investigations are needed. The suicidal or homicidal risks, if any, are assessed as well as the use or abuse of drugs which complicates the disease or treatment plan are revealed. The patient's motivation to abstain from the substance abuse, his co-operation, medical compliance as well as his resources (financial and also social support) are also areas which can be, at least minimally, assessed during the interview. The interview should reveal the nature, course and chronicity of the illness and help the physician to reach a working diagnosis, because only after this the future therapeutic programme can be chalked out and any possible prediction made regarding the outcome of the disease.

The interview subserves yet another important function. It helps to develop a good working relationship termed rapport with the patient. Good rapport is essential to gather data particularly in sensitive areas of patient's life which are often vital in reaching a diagnosis. The interview further motivates the patient and aids the curative process. Medical technology

1

has advanced considerably and the tools for investigation are more powerful and refined which aid more precise conclusions. But these in no way minimize the importance of clinical interview by which a clinician can evaluate the symptoms and signs more methodically in the context of patient's cultural milieu.

Of the various tools of examination available, conversation is the oldest and the most important. With its adaptation to a clinical setting the clinician relies on no method as heavily as the interview to know about the patient and his complaints. The ability to conduct it with scientific precision and thoroughness and at the same time with an artistic sensitivity without offending the patient is the psychiatrist's skill which comes only after long years of practice. During this process the interviewer has to meet many challenges. The uniqueness and individuality of each patient have to be taken into account, being aware at the same time of the educational and sociocultural milieu in which the patient lives. The reliability of the presented data has to be assessed and checked. Indirect methods of eliciting history or examination have to be devised when the patient becomes 'non-cooperative'. Above all, the therapeutic rapport which was established has to be maintained with the patient till the end leading to a successful completion of the examination.

## DEVELOPMENT OF RAPPORT

Rapport is the harmonious relationship which the patient develops with his therapist in the course of treatment.

The doctor works with diseased people, not with a bunch of disease syndromes. "There are no diseases—only sick people". Patients come with a rainbow of emotional display—anxiety, fear, sorrow or even hostility and resentment. The doctor who is successful in gaining their confidence and allaying their anxiety prepares the soil for a good therapeutic alliance. The patient reposes his trust in the doctor whom he accepts as one who knows and understands him. This is the beginning of building up a good rapport and the step stone to a successful doctor–patient relationship. Having a good rapport is essential in any clinical setting not only in psychiatry but also in any branch of medicine.

Some interview skills and techniques are helpful in creating and maintaining a good rapport.

1. Conduct the interview in a quiet place with least external disturbance and distractions and where privacy is ensured.

2. Adopt an unhurried and relaxed pose throughout the interview. Maintain eye contact with the patient.

3. Listen attentively to what the patient says. Do not assume a bored, indifferent or skeptical attitude.

4. Encourage patient in his narration by making occasional facilitatory remarks or by nonverbal expressions of assurance and concern.

5. Pick up cues of distress or other intense emotional turmoil in the patient and pursue them in the conversation. This is empathizing or sharing what the patient experiences.

6. Avoid interruptions and distractions as much as possible.

7. When the patient digresses from the theme or loses his track, guide him to the main theme politely.

8. While taking notes be as unobtrusive as possible without interfering with the conversation.

9. Avoid antagonising remarks and value judgements.

10. Do not offer premature conclusions and assurances on the outcome of treatment.

11. Avoid unduly prolonging the interview. Interviews should not ordinarily be stretched beyond 40–50 minutes. In special situations interviews will have to be cut much shorter.

One of the most important considerations in an interview setting is privacy to ensure free exchange of ideas and confidentiality. A quiet place away from the chattering of the curious onlookers is necessary. Bedside consultation in a busy general ward is not an ideal place for psychiatric interview because of the above reasons. Vital information which a patient is otherwise ready to divulge may be held back if the environment is not conducive for a free talk. The doctor's assurance that the information thus accessed will be kept confidential aids communication.

Even though privacy is ideal and a number of patients do not want the presence of relatives, there are situations which warrant against the interviewer to be alone with the patient. Patients who are violent and aggressive or psychotics who exhibit out-of-control behaviour are best interviewed along with a relative against whom the patient is not hostile. Safety, both for the patient and the doctor, is to be ensured during the interview. Security staff should be available for help if needed, and the patient is ideally searched for hidden weapons. The doctor should be seated in such a way that he has a free access to the exit door.

## TYPES OF INTERVIEW

Broadly there are three methods of conducting the interview. In the 'free' type, the interviewer assumes the role of a listener without trying to direct the course of the interview. He asks open or sometimes leading questions and thereafter says as little as possible except by way of encouragement to the patient to proceed further. If there are pauses, the interviewer repeats the last words of the patient. Once the patient starts talking he keeps him going, occasionally asking him to elaborate a particular detail. The advantages of this technique is that it is least threatening to the former. There is no danger of the doctor monopolising the interview and of implanting his own ideas and speculations in the patient's mind. A unique advantage of this type of interview is that it gives a wealth of unexpected information which the other types do not provide. What the patient says and how he says will give clues to the doctor on what to ask him further and how. But if not guided properly the interview drags and deteriorates into a social conversation and obtaining a chaos of often unimportant details with the main themes being left untouched. There is also the danger of patient dominating the interview.

In the second type called the 'directed interview'— the physician deciding on the grounds which he wants to cover asks more direct questions. For example, instead of asking about the family environment in general he might specifically ask about the attitude of the patient towards his father. This method has the advantage over the free type in that it covers a number of important areas. However, it is uncomfortable to the patient and puts him on guard. Also, some areas are left untouched which, though important to the patient, are missed by the interviewer. The patient has only a passive role and may not be an active participant.

In the third type called the 'structured interview' or the 'questionnaire method', the interviewer prepares a set of standard questions which are administered to all his patients alike, generally in the same order. Like the former this method is also disturbing to the patient. The method brings forth a mass of details which are however flat and colourless without any emotional contours. Other limitations of this type are that it does not reveal all information which the patient might otherwise volunteer. The patient may even deny, or falsify some statements either willfully or by not understanding the questions put to him. Though primarily used for research purposes this method is also used in clinical interviews. Overdependence on the questionnaire method only helps to pigeonhole the clinical material into a few rigid categories.

All the three techniques can be judiciously combined in the same interview with advantage. As the details start emerging they are fitted in the conceptual framework of a questionnaire which the interviewer, in his mind should have prepared beforehand. Missing details are added later on by direct questioning. Thus beginning with a free type the interview winds up in a more direct manner and ends with a brief structured session to fill any gaps left uncovered.

Suggestive and leading questions which are usually held invalid in clinical interviews have an important role in psychiatry. These are questions which suggest their own answers and in general should be avoided. But there are instances where their use is warranted and where they can be used without fear of suggesting the answers—as in schizo-phrenia, while enquiring about the perceptual abnormalities. Though decried as a risky tool their use in a differential manner can be advantageous.

The setting of the interview is very crucial. Privacy and confidentiality are essential factors as well as comfort to the patient but the most vital part of the setting is provided by the interviewer himself, by his genuine unaffected interest in the patient. The physician should maintain a necessary objectivity and detachment which should be distinguished from scientific aloofness and negligence. From such a position the physician can remain patient, tolerant and sufficiently free from personal anxiety aroused by unwarranted flattery or hostile rebuff from the patient's side.

## LIMIT SETTING IN PSYCHIATRY

Often interview techniques will have to be tailored to suit certain special clinical situations. This is dealt in a subsequent chapter on patients posing special problems. Among them a particular group of patients need special mention who by their dominating behaviour restrict the doctor's freedom and set their own conditions of treatment. The doctor should be watchful for such behaviour which may present as noncompliance to the permitted time limits, throwing temper tantrums, destructiveness or violence. The doctor should thwart such attempts by specifying which behaviour qualitatively and quantitatively will be acceptable from the patient and which will not. This may be done verbally (by verbally disapproving it) or behaviourally (e.g. not responding to the inappropriate piece of behaviour). This is limit setting which has a crucial role in any interview set ups.

If the patient is accompanied by a relative, it is preferable to see the patient first. In many cases this will allay the patient's fears and anxiety that the doctor is influenced by his hostile family members to act as their accomplice in persecuting him. But the patient should be informed of the necessity of seeing the relative also for additional information. Besides providing additional information this would also help to uncover the relative's attitude to the patient and his illness which might as well be unhealthy, such as overprotective, demanding, unrealistic, intolerant or outright condemning.

While the interview is in progress the examiner should not enter into arguments with the patient. The results not only are nonprofitable but are also damaging and the interviewer will soon realise that the hard earned rapport is lost within no time often irrecoverably. He should not dub the details provided by the patient as unimportant or false and also should avoid pointing out inconsistencies, thereby embarassing the patient. Patients agree to participate in the interview with a desire to be understood and for an appreciative response from the examiner. If the patient discovers that both of these are lacking, he would not like to continue attending the sessions.

Often patients are come across who require no special prodding for volunteering information. The stimulus of a receptive environment is more than enough for them to verbalise their complaints and about themselves unendingly, unless the interviewer is able to divert the stream of talk gainfully. A novice untrained to pick up the facts from such a jumble would be tempted to call this as 'irrelevant talk', though a study of the patient's frame of mind helps to reveal its hidden relevance to him. Often the abundant details are aimed at self-justification. As is correctly said the 'irrelevance' is merely a condition of the interviewer's mind, when he does not know what to make of the patient's talk.

Almost invariably the interview begins with the presenting problems of the patient. This has the advantage of being a topic which is of serious mutual interest to both the patient and the doctor and it is likely to be the topic on which the patient is ready to talk spontaneously. To know why the patient chose to come to the hospital provides the soundest basis for the interviewer also to start the conversation. It is important to record verbatim the words of the patient as and where he describes his symptoms. Attempts to translate his words and descriptions into another language might result in dilution or even distortion of their meaning. The patient's attitude towards his symptoms and illness in general would be reflected in his words, which again would be lost in the process of translation. The interviewer should not attach his own meanings and interpretations while recording the symptoms.

The next topic which logically would follow will be the history of present illness. This is the gradual unfolding of his symptoms from the earliest time at which a change was noticed by the patient, till his arrival in the hospital. The interviewer should enquire whether everything had been going well up to this time, and also the circumstances which led to his coming now. The manner of patient's narration is again important though this has necessarily to be condensed to suit the records.

It is not the purpose of this chapter to go into a detailed schema of history taking. This is dealt in the next chapter on history taking and examination. It is however worthwhile to emphasise that the value of the record lies in the wealth of data explored and collected. The history is not a collection of scattered events. It is the record of development and unfurling of his symptoms in step with the patient's life events and adjustment and reaction to them. The value of the examination lies in discovering the relevance of the events to the development of the present illness.

The history provides a longitudinal account of the patient's symptoms. What is further required is a cross-sectional analysis of his behaviour and an exposition of his subjective mode of experience. This is done during the mental status examination through which the examiner reaches a phenomenological clarity of the patient's symptoms. It does not mean that the mental status examination has to wait till the history taking is over. In fact, it starts as soon as the patient enters the consultation room and goes hand in hand with the interview from the observation of his general behaviour, prevailing mood, style and tempo of talk, intelligent presentation of symptoms, etc. Whatever is left out or is hidden from the general scrutiny of areas which require further elaboration is kept to the last and tested in detail in a manner described in the following chapters.

Accurate, consistent and reliable clinical recording is absolutely essential, not only for making the records research-worthy, but also for good care of the patients. The main purposes of good recordkeeping are:

1. Identification of patients and their illnesses.
2. Knowing the up-to-date status of the patient
3. Aiding communication.
4. Reporting to other agencies and referral sources.
5. Statistical purposes
6. Epidemiological studies
7. Legal purposes

Under these broad goals a variety of subsidiary aims and uses can be subsumed.

While flexibility is advantageous during the examination of a patient, recording is best done in accordance with a definite schema. Obsessive adherence to a schema during the examination and drilling the patient for information on each point provoke resentment and irritation in him; whereas non-compliance to schema during recording will result in disorderliness and scattering of data, when the examiner will have to hunt for the misplaced details all throughout the pages of the case sheet.

The various tasks in front of the clinician have been well narrated by another author and are the following:

1. Outline the goals of interview;
2. Establish rapport;
3. Be empathetic, not sympathetic. Try to evaluate the symptoms from the patient's perspective;
4. Enforce limit setting;
5. Communicate clearly and in simple non-technical language;
6. Assess mental status and collect pertinent data while in conversation with the patient;
7. Check reliability of data obtained from patient and others—understand the possibility of subjective colouring of details;
8. Assess suicidal and homicidal risks of the patient as well as the risks of violence and aggression and those due to co-existing medical conditions;
9. Collect collateral information;
10. Document all details.

## FURTHER READING

1. Andrews Linda B. The Psychiatric Interview and Mental Status Examination. In: Robert E Hales, Stuart C Yudofsky and Glen O Gabbard (eds). Textbook of Psychiatry, 5th ed. American Psychiatric Publishing Inc (2008).

2. Gelder M, Gath D, May on R, Cowen P. Interviewing, Clinical examination and record keeping. In: Oxford Textbook of Psychiatry, 3rd ed. Oxford, 1996.

3. Ripley HS. The Psychiatric Examination. In: Freedman AM, Kaplan HI, eds. Comprehensive Textbook of Psychiatry. Williams and Wilkins, 1967.

4. Strauss GD. The Psychiatric interview, history and mental status examination. In: Kaplan HI, Saddock BJ, eds. Comprehensive Textbook of Psychiatry, 6th ed. Williams and Wilkins, 1995.

# 2

# History Taking and Examination

VMD Namboodiri, TP Subhalakshmi

## INTRODUCTION

A detailed and reliable history usually elicited from patient, his relatives and close friends and documented chronologically is of supreme importance in any branch of medicine. In psychiatry its value is exceptional. While there is no one correct method of eliciting and recording the history, it is necessary for the trainee to be adept in one standard form so as to ensure that all areas are covered and that no details are left out. A conventional form is presented in this chapter which preferably is gone through routinely till one becomes proficient and selective and understands that all questions are not needed in all instances.

History should be collected from other reliable sources also, as not seldom, the patient may not be able to or want to give all details related to his complaints or disturbed functions. History thus obtained from collateral sources should not be mixed with patient's descriptions but should be recorded separately.

History may be collected and recorded under the following arbitrary heads:

1. Identification data and demographical details.
2. Presenting complaints.
3. History of present illness.
4. History of past psychiatric illness.
5. Family history.
6. Psychosocial history.

11

7. Personal history.
8. Premorbid personality.
9. Medical history.

## Scheme of History Taking

### 1. Identification of Demographic Details

This should include the patient's name and address, age, gender, religion, socioeconomic status, hospital number, marital status, occupation and source of referral as well as details of the informant. The latter should include name of the informant, relation to the patient, intimacy and length of acquaintance and the interviewer's impression on the reliability of the information provided by him.

### 2. Presenting Complaints and Duration

As mentioned in the previous chapter patients would often like to talk starting with their complaints. While recording them always use simple and non-technical language. It is customary to record the patient's words verbatim without paraphrasing or interpreting them. The opening words of the patient are important and give an insight into the patient's own judgement of his symptoms and their relative importance as perceived by him. Often patients deny of having any complaints and say that they were forcibly brought to the hospital by hostile relatives. In such cases this should be recorded. Denial of illness need not always point to a lack of insight and might account for various social pressures.

Attempts should be made to note the severity and duration of each symptom. If the patient or his relatives are unable to tell the time relations, they may be asked when the patient was last seen well and asymptomatic. Or find out whether they could link the onset to any important personal, family or social event.

After the patient voluntarily states his symptoms, it would be worthwhile to ask him whether he has or had any other symptom other than those disclosed by him.

### 3. Mode of Onset and Progression

The complaints may have a sudden onset of a few days duration when the onset is described as acute or sudden. However, in many instances the patient or informant may not be able to give a definite time relation to the onset of behavioural changes-which in a subtle and unnoticeable manner had been persisting over months or years. The onset is then described as insidious. As in other medical conditions, in psychiatry also the course of symptoms could be steady and progressive, diminishing and reappearing periodically, remitting and relapsing at regular intervals (cyclical) or staying in the same way over the time.

## 4. Precipitating Factors

Very often some events or factors are alluded as precipitants to the illness by the patient or relatives. Though cause and effect cannot be established with certainty and the described precipitants could be merely coincidental, these events as well as other specific stressors which occurred antecedental to the onset of illness are to be taken into consideration. The temporal relations, severity of stressors, patient's preoccupation with them, and the personal value attached to the events may all give a clue to the presence and nature of the precipitant. The interviewer should also be aware of the influence of culture on phenomenology and the attributed precipitating factors. This is dealt in more detail in a subsequent chapter.

## 5. History of Present Illness

This is a chronological unfolding of the patient's symptoms from the time they were first noted to their present status along with patient's reactions to them. The patient should be allowed to narrate the history in his own words without interruption and without making him feel embarrassed in any way. Enquire about each symptom individually—its severity, duration, progression and also the temporal association with other symptoms. Correlate them with significant life events of the patient like death in the family, financial setbacks, shifting of residence, change of jobs, concurrent illness, etc. Ask about their impact on patient's emotional, sexual, marital, family, work and social domains and life functioning in general. It is often useful and informative to make the patient or the informant describe a typical day in the patient's life after becoming ill. Ask about the biological functions like sleep, appetite, change in weight, bowel and bladder habits, libido, diurnal variation in symptoms, etc. Take a detailed negative history to rule out other diagnoses—organic, substance related and other functional psychiatric disorders. Enquire about any treatment taken, adherence to treatment and the effect of treatment on the symptoms.

Patient's history may have to be supplemented with data provided by the informant particularly when the former is deficient or when the patient, because of his illness, is unable to give a coherent account. History provided by the patient or the informant may have gaps which should be filled up by carefully selected leading questions on the missing details. When the patient has finished speaking spontaneously, the interviewer should summarize the problems that have been mentioned, and ask if there are any others.

At the end of the exercise the interviewer should have a detailed, coherent and chronological account of the patient's illness from the earliest time a change was noted to the time of presentation to the examiner.

### 6. History of Past Psychiatric Illness

Enquire whether the patient has had any psychiatric illness in the past; its nature, duration, course, treatment and response, hospitalizations and patient's adherence to treatment.

### 7. Family History

This should include consanguinity, details of the size and type (nuclear, extended or joint) of the family and the number of people living together. Since the family is the immediate social environment of the patient, details of all important persons as the parents, siblings, etc. should be gone into individually. Enquire about the general family environment. Is it harmonious? Are there frequent quarrels in the family?

Presence of psychiatric illness, alcohol or other substance use, suicide, personality problems, seizure disorder, intellectual disability, dementia, etc. in the family should be routinely enquired about. A positive history might indicate a hereditary basis for the patient's illness. Family data are important in other ways also. Family in no small measure moulds one's personality and stresses in the family might precipitate a psychiatric illness. Conversely, a happy family will be conducive to treatment and enhances a patient's recovery.

## 8. Social Circumstances

The social environment to which the patient and family are exposed may play a role in the patient's illness in the causation, maintenance or management. Focus on the social support available to the patient and family.

## 9. Personal History

The personal history includes the developmental of the history, educational and occupational history, and the sexual and marital history of the individual and constitutes a significant area in history taking.

### a. Developmental History

Early development: Enquire about details of pregnancy—whether pregnancy was planned or not; parents' attitude to the birth of the child; gender preferences; attempt to abort; mother's health during pregnancy; illnesses and use of drugs; nature of delivery and complications if any; birth defects and parents' attitude to them; habit training difficulties if any, and developmental milestones (sitting, standing, walking, sphincter control, speech, etc.); health as an infant and medications; whether precocious or retarded in growth; 'neurotic traits' if any as tantrums, thumb sucking and nail biting, fears, food fads, stammering, nocturnal enuresis, mannerisms.

Childhood and adolescence: Health, medications and hospitalizations, entry to school, relationship with teachers and peers; truancy and other deviant behaviour; dreams and fantasies; ambitions; relationship with parents and other authority figures; reaction to stress and frustrations; group activities (leader or follower?), perseverance; significant happenings as a child—particularly death of close relatives, separation, etc.

Adulthood and later life: Employment, marriage and settling in life; deviant behaviour if any; significant events in life.

### b. Educational and Work History

These areas touched upon briefly in the previous section should be elaborated here.

Education: Age of starting and finishing; types of schools; academic records; games and sports; hobbies and interests;

nicknames; special abilities, disabilities and achievements; extent of educational failures. It may be useful to note down if there is any gross disparity in patient's educational achievements when compared to that of his siblings.

Occupation: Chronological list of jobs held with reasons for change; present occupation; job satisfaction and dissatisfaction if any and cause; work record.

## c. Sexual History

Menstrual history: Age at menarche, regularity of periods, premenstrual tension; age of menopause and symptoms associated with menopause, if any.

Sexual practices: Attitude towards sex; masturbation; guilt feelings; homosexual and heterosexual experience prior to and after marriage; perversions, if any.

Marital history: Age at marriage; arranged or not? Was the marriage forced by pregnancy or other compelling circumstances? Age, health, occupation and personality of spouse; contraceptive measures; quarrels, separations.

Children: Age, name and sex; miscarriages; parent's attitude to children.

## 10. Premorbid Personality

An attempt should be made to know what type of person he was prior to illness and his strengths and weaknesses. Observation during the interview might give some clues. Information though coloured subjective and personal biases is however largely obtained from patient's own description of himself and from other people's accounts. Descriptive examples of patient's behaviour at selected situations will often provide rich and useful data.

a. *Social relations:* Does he have many friends or only a few? Own sex or opposite sex? Of the same age or much older or younger? Relation with colleagues and workmates; membership in club and societies; whether friendship is deep or superficial? Does he change friends too often?
b. *Use of leisure time:* Hobbies and interests
c. *Mood and general disposition:* Anxious, cheerful, despondent, distrustful? Does his mood fluctuate without any reason?

d. *Character:* Sensitive, suspicious, resentful, quarrelsome, shy, reserved, self critical, boisterous?

e. *Standards:* Moral, religious and health standards; ambitions; perfectionistic; level of aspiration.

f. *Habit:* Food, sleep and excretory functions: use of alcohol or other substances.

g. *Level of energy:* Level of initiative, energetic, sluggish, perseverance.

## 11. Medical History

This as well as the past psychiatric history may be included in the personal history but are considered separately here because of their unique importance. History of past or concurrent physical illness, accidents particularly head injuries, hospitalizations and surgical interventions should be gained as well as details of any medicines which patient currently takes.

## MENTAL STATE EXAMINATION (MSE)

The mental state is concerned with the symptoms and behaviour at the time of the interview. It is a cross-sectional picture of a patient's functioning. There is a degree of overlap between the history and the mental state. The order of the elements of the MSE given below does not imply a sequence that must be followed. The interviewing clinician should adopt a sequence that encourages the flow of information that is responsive to the patient's affect and condition.

Different aspects of psychopathology are discussed in detail in the subsequent chapters. Only an outline of the MSE along with possible facilitating questions are given below.

### 1. Appearance, behaviour and attitude

Make systematic notes about the patient's appearance, behaviour and attitude to the examiner.

### Appearance

Body build: Short/tall; thin/overweight; any appearance suggesting recent weight loss as in physical illness, depression, chronic anxiety.

Posture: Depressed patient sits with head inclined downwards, anxious patient with head erect but often on the edge of the chair with hands gripping its sides.

Clothes, grooming, hygiene: Does the patient appear appropriately dressed and clean/ dirty unkempt looks (possibilities include alcohol dependence, substance abuse, depression, dementia, schizophrenia); manic patients may wear bright colours, adopt incongruous styles of dress or appear poorly groomed; does the patient appear dishevelled or meticulous; does the patient look ill?

Facial appearance: Depressed patient—turning down of the corners of the mouth, vertical furrows on the brow, and a slight raising of the medial aspect of each brow; anxious patients may show horizontal creases on the forehead, raised eyebrows, widened palpebral fissures, dilated pupils, unchanging 'wooden' expression of patients taking drugs with Parkinsonian side effects.

### Psychomotor Behaviour

It includes all nonverbal behaviour by the patient during the interview. This section of the MSE must be complemented by a thorough neurological examination to clarify any suspicious findings.

Gait: Note how the patient walks (e.g. ataxia, broad-based, festinating)

Level of activity: Hyperactive, agitated, combative, akathisia, fidgety, retarded.

Movements: Clumsy, agile, rigid.

Look for:
- Gestures
- Tics
- Mannerism
- Stereotypies
- Echopraxia
- Waxy flexibility
- Extra-pyramidal symptoms
- Negativism
- Ambitendence
- Tardive dyskinesia
- Akathisia

## Interpersonal Behaviour and Attitude Towards Examiner

Manic patients often show over familiarity. Schizophrenics may be overactive, withdrawn or aggressive. Demented patients may respond unconventionally or may sit preoccupied. In recording abnormal social behaviour, give a clear description of what the patient actually does:

- Cooperative/non-cooperative
- Attentive/interested/frank
- Guarded/evasive/defensive/suspicious/hostile/threatens violence
- Poised/submissive
- Ill at ease/self critical
- Contemptuous/manipulative

## Level of Rapport

Establishing a relationship is essential for obtaining history and assessing psychopathology. Unless a trusting relationship has been established, patients will not reveal the personal, intimate, and diagnostically important details of their experience. Note down whether you are able to establish a rapport with the patient.

Eye contact: Can the patient make and tolerate eye contact or does he seeks to avoid it?

## 2. Cognitive Status

### Sensorium

The patient's level of arousal and attention are evaluated by observation and testing. Levels of hypoarousal vary from drowsiness to stupor and coma. Does the patient appear to be in reasonable touch with his surroundings and responsive to external stimuli?

- Comatose – state of unarousable unresponsiveness
- Stuporous – needs vigorous stimulation to be aroused
- Drowsy – patient is fatigued and falls asleep when unstimulated
- Alert
- Hypervigilant

## Attention and Concentration

Attention is the ability to focus on the matter in hand and concentration is the ability to sustain that focus. Attention is impaired in disorders of arousal but may also be abnormal in patients who are fully alert. Is the patient able to maintain his attention or does he appear to be easily diverted or distracted? If distractible, is there any reason for this? Digit span test, serial subtraction test (e.g. serial sevens test), spelling words backwards, reverse digit span, reciting the days of the week or the months of the year in reverse order. Both accuracy and speed of performance are observed.

- Attention easily aroused and sustained/distractible
- Concentration

### Orientation

This is assessed by asking about the patient's awareness of person, place, time and social context. If the patient cannot answer these questions correctly, he should be asked about his own identity.

Person

Place

Time:

- day
- date
- month
- year

Social context

### Memory

Memory can be assessed in both verbal and non-verbal domains. Inquiring about personal orientation is one means of assessing recent memory. Registration and immediate memory are assessed by asking the patient to repeat sequences of digits that have been spoken slowly enough for him to register them with reasonable expectation. Word-list memory tests may be given for assessing learning, recall and recognition. The patient is given three words to remember and then is asked to recall them three minutes later. The examiner notes how much difficulty the patient has in learning the three words initially and how many times the words must be presented before the patient can repeat all the three. If the patient cannot remember the words after a few minutes, the patient is given clues. This helps to distinguish between storage and recall deficits. Remote memory is tested by asking about the patient's significant life events (dates of graduation, marriage, birth dates of children) and by asking about political leaders and important historical events.

- Immediate memory
- Recent memory
- Remote memory
- Effect of defect on patient
- Attitude towards deficit

### General Information and Intelligence

In most clinical interviews, intelligence is inferred rather than tested specifically. Questions should have some relevance to the patient's educational and cultural background. Note down

- Patient's level of formal education and self education
- Estimate of the patient's intellectual capacity (assess patient's vocabulary, ability to interpret proverbs, make him or her do calculations)
- General knowledge

### 3. Mood

Check how the patient is feeling by asking "What is your mood like?" "How are you feeling in your spirits at the moment?" When enquiry about mood indicates depression, it is mandatory that the interviewer looks for other features which may suggest a high suicidal risk.

Subjective: The patient's own assessment of his mood

Objective: Observed or described by others

Adjectival description of the predominant mood:

- Calm
- Depressed
- Irritable
- Anxious

- Fearful
- Terrified
- Angry
- Happy
- Elated
- Euphoric
- Apathetic

Intensity / depth

### Range

Reactivity: The fluctuations in mood that occur in parallel with changes to one's environment. Monotonic / labile: When mood varies excessively, it is said to be labile. For example, the patient appears dejected at one point in the interview but quickly changes to a normal or unduly cheerful mood. Any persisting lack of affect, usually called a blunting or flattening, should be noted.

Appropriateness and Congruity: Some discuss inappropriateness in relation to the situations and incongruity to ideation level. Check whether the patient's professed mood fits with what he has been saying.

Abnormal emotional reactions are those that are understandable but excessive. In abnormal expression of emotions there is qualitative or experiential difference from the average normal reaction; however, the person is aware of the abnormality. In morbid disorders of emotional expression, on the other hand, the person is unaware of the abnormality, e.g. a patient cheerfully telling the examiner that he has been asked by voices to murder his relatives.

Infectivity
Somatic accompaniments
Ideas of suicide

### 4. Perception

Enquiries should be made tactfully, without making the patient feel offended. Commonsense judgement is needed to decide when it is safe to omit such enquiries altogether. Questions can be introduced by saying, "Have you ever had any unusual experiences like hearing sounds or voices when no one else is within earshot?" Find out whether the patient has heard a single voice or several; if the latter, whether the voices appear to talk to each other about the patient in the third person or voices speaking to him (second person).

### Sensory Distortions

1. Changes in intensity
2. Changes in quality
3. Changes in spatial form
4. Body image distortions

### Sensory Deceptions

1. Illusions
2. Hallucinations (find out the content, circumstances of occurrence):
   a. Hallucinations of individual senses
      * Hearing
      * Vision
      * Smell
      * Touch
      * Taste
      * Pain and deep sensations
      * Vestibular sensations
   b. Special kinds of hallucinations
      * Functional hallucinations
      * Reflex hallucinations
      * Extracampine hallucinations
      * Autoscopy

### Other Perceptual Experiences

1. Depersonalization
2. Derealisation
3. Déjà vu

4. Jamais vu

5. Macropsia

6. Micropsia

The patient's attitude to perceptual disturbances.

## 5. Speech

How the patient speaks is recorded under this heading, whereas what he/she says is recorded under disorders of thought.

If the patient is mute, test ability to produce sounds and communicate non-verbally.

Reaction time: Slow/quick (does the patient's reply come immediately or is it delayed?)

Spontaneity: Spontaneous/nonspontaneous (patient speaks only when asked something)/hesitant/mute.

Productivity: Monosyllabic/elaborate

Pitch: Monotonous/whispered/loud

Speed: Fast/slow

Articulation

• Slurring

• Stammering

• Dysarthria

**Anything notable about:**

• Vocabulary

• Choice of words

Record a sample of conversation/speech/talk for a detailed analysis.

## 6. Thinking

From the quality of speech and writings the interviewer makes inferences about the processes of thinking and cognitive organization.

### *Stream*

• Flight of ideas

• Retardation

- Circumstantiality
- Thought blocking

## Form

- Poverty of thought
- Poverty of content of thought
- Tangentiality
- Derailment
- Incoherence
- Illogicality
- Clang associations
- Neologism
- Word approximation
- Echolalia
- Stilted speech
- Self reference
- Paraphasia
- Stereotypy
- Perseveration
- Concreteness
- Overinclusiveness

## Possession

Obsessions and compulsions: Do any thoughts, ideas, doubts, images, impulses keep coming into your mind, even though you try hard not to have them? If the answer is 'yes', ask for an example. Do you have to do things over and over again when most people would have done them only once? Give example(s).

Thought alienaton(insertion, withdrawal, broadcasting)

## Content

1. Preoccupations: About the illness/environmental problems/ depressive ideas/phobias/hypochondriacal symptoms.
2. Delusions

- Types according to onset
  Primary/secondary
- Types according to theme
  Persecution/love/jealousy/grandeur/ill health/guilt/nihilism/poverty
- Other features
  Mood congruent/incongruent
  Systematization
  Shared delusions

## 7. Abstract Thinking

Disturbance in concept formation; manner in which the patient conceptualizes or handles ideas; similarities and differences; absurdities; meanings of simple proverbs; answers may be concrete (giving specific examples to illustrate the meaning), overly abstract (giving general explanations).

Appropriateness of answers should be noted.

## 8. Insight

Degree of awareness and understanding the patient has that he or she is ill.

- Degree
- Anosognosia
- Psychogenic anosognosia
- Labelle indifference

## 9. Judgement

- Personal judgement
- Social judgement
- Test judgement

## PHYSICAL EXAMINATION

The examination of the patient is not complete without a physical examination. Even when the patient is referred to you by another specialist, it is always safer to do a general physical examination. The timing and the extent of the examination is decided by considering the diagnostic possibilities in the individual case. When there is doubt, a systematic physical examination should be performed, and should include a careful examination of the endocrine and nervous systems. A female patient should be examined in the presence of a female attendant, if the examiner is a male. Look also for possession of harmful substances and objects.

# 3

# Disturbances of Motor Behaviour

Rajat Ray, Ravi Gupta

## INTRODUCTION

Though the term "disturbance of motor disorders" classically depicts the abnormal involuntary movements and is considered primarily the area of neurology, they are not uncommon among psychiatric patients. One of the reasons is the common substrate for the development of such a disorder is the brain. The brain is regulating behaviour including the sensory-motor aspects, hence, any abnormality in the substrate of brain, behavioural as well as sensory-motor symptoms can be observed.

Contrary to the classical depiction of "movement disorders" as is seen in Neurology, the term "disturbance of motor behaviour" in this chapter would describe the abnormal movements seen across a variety of psychiatric disorders. Broadly speaking, abnormal movements seen among psychiatric patients canbe divided intoan increment of activity and a reduction in the activity as compared to the normal level of activity.

This chapter would discuss the following conditions briefly.

1. **Simple Non-purposive/Quasi-purposive Hyperkinetic Movement Disorders:** These include tremors, dyskinesia, dystonia, tics and myoclonus. During these movements, only one muscle or a small set of muscles is involved and they do not simulate any complex movement.

   a. **Tremors:** Tremors are defined as the repetitive movements that arise because of alternate contraction of the agonists and antagonists muscles.

29

b. **Dyskinisia:** These are non-goal directed movements that usually involve the bucco-facial muscles or the fingers or the toes. They are involuntary in nature but may be abolished for some time at will. Common dyskinisias are lip-smacking, puckering, tongue-protrusion, chewing or mastication, foot tapping or finger tapping.

c. **Dystonia:** It manifests as altered tone of muscles where it remains in the state of contraction causing altered posture but without repetitive movements as seen by the above-mentioned categories.

d. **Tics:** Tics are the sudden, repetitive movements that are involuntary but can be stopped temporarily at will. Common tics are frowning, shoulder shrugging, jerking the neck.

e. **Myoclonus:** Myoclonus is defined as sudden jerky movement lasting for a second or so. Myoclonic movements can be seen during myoclonic epilepsy. It can also be encountered in at the transition of wakefulness to sleep.

2. **Complex Quasi-purposive/Purposeful Hyperkinetic Movement Disorders:**

a. These movements are termed complex because they often involve more than one muscle group and are done to accomplish some act. Among psychiatric patients, purposeful movements are seen which can be completely voluntary, semi-voluntary or involuntary. Voluntary complex purposeful movements are seen during aggression; semi-voluntary when the patient has partial control over it, as seen during compulsive touching in obsessive compulsive disorder (OCD) or akathisia, children with Attention-Deficit/Hyperactivity Disorder (ADHD) and anxiety.

b. **Complex voluntary purposeful movements:** These movements may be seen during the episodes of schizophrenia or bipolar disorder and are aimed at protecting oneself by acting on the delusions or hallucinations. These movements are rarely premeditated as we see with criminal acts but are often impulsive.

c. **Complex involuntary semi-purposeful movements:** Chorea is repetitive, jerky movements that traverse from one part of the body to another. Sometimes patients try to include these movements into some kind of purposeful activity thus, they appear quasi-purposive.

3. **Hypokinetic Movement Disorders:** While the excessive movements are the cause of clinical concern, at the same time, a reduction or absence of movements can also evoke worries. In psychiatry, these symptoms may represent an illness (catatonia) or at other times, they may represent the adverse effect of medications (drug induced Parkinson's).

Disturbance in motor behaviour

- **Simple non-purposive hyperkinetic movement**
- **Simple quasi-purposive hyperkinetic movement**
- **Complex non-purposive hyperkinetic movement**
- **Complex quasi-purposive hyperkinetic movement**
- **Hypokinetic movement**

Furthermore, such disorders (disturbance of motor behaviour) can be seen:

- As a part of neurodevelopment disorder seen among children and adolescents
- As a part of psychiatric diseases as catatonia
- As drug side effects or medication induced
- Sleep related disorders
- Catatonia seen among a number of medical conditions

The chapter would focus on these themes and as relevant in clinical psychiatry along with an outline of management.

### a. Population—Children and Adolescents

Children as a part of *Autism Spectrum Disorder* may display not well coordinated motor performance which interferes with activities of daily living. These include repetitive apparently purposeless motor behaviour such as hand shaking, waving, body rocking, head banging, etc. A **tic** is a sudden rapid recurrent non-rhythmic motor movement of vocalisation.

Certain abnormal motor behaviour is also seen among subjects with *Attention-Deficit/Hyperactivity Disorder (ADHD)*. Such patients display:

- Task inattention
- Easy distractibility
- Fidgety behaviour
- Unable to remain quiet
- Hyperactive
- Impulsive behaviour

### b. Psychiatric Illness—Schizophrenia Spectrum and Other Psychotic Disorders

These patients would need to fulfil the criteria to establish the diagnosis of schizophrenia and as additional features/ modifiers display catatonic features.

Catatonia usually describes a state of stupor, immobility, or a state of chaotic physical and psychological agitation.

The features of catatonia are:

- Marked psychomotor retardation sometimes complete immobility
- Waxy flexibility (no resistance from the patients while the examiner is attempting to move the limb)
- Excitement
- Negativism (strong opposition to whatever is being done or attempted)
- Peculiar voluntary movements like posturing, mannerism, grimacing, etc.
- Mutism
- Echolalia (repeating the examiner's speech)
- Echopraxia (repeating the examiner's movement or behaviour)
- Refusal to eat or drink

These are to be observed during mental state examination (MSE) as a part of examination of appearance and behaviour. More specifically motor activity can be noted as either bradykinesia or hyperkinesias. On occasions these are also observed during neuropsychological examination. Here motor assessment would include handedness, ability to carry out large motor tasks and provide information on attention, executive functions and sensory/motor functioning.

Besides *Schizophrenia,* stupor can be seen in *Affective Illness* and (rarely) as *Hysterical Catatonia.* Furthermore, disturbance of motor behaviour including catatonia can be seen in (to name some conditions):

- Autism (described earlier)
- A number of medical conditions
- Subarachnoid haemorrhages
- Basal ganglion disorders
- Endocrine and metabolic disorders
- Locked-in and akinetic-mutism state
- Dementia
- Drug induced

### c. Medication Induced

Most common movement disorders reported have been parkinsonism, acute dystonia and acute akithisia. Nueroleptic-malignant syndrome is a life threatening situation in psychiatry. The introduction of newer anti-psychotic drugs has greatly reduced the incidence of extra pyramidal side effects and medication induced movement disorders. However, medication like *olanzepine, aripiprazole* and in rare instance antidepressants like *antidepressants (Selective Serotonin Reuptake Inhibitors-SSRI)* can cause akathisia and dyskinisia.

**Medications likely to cause high occurrence of movement disorders**

- **Fluphenazine**
- **Haloperidol**
- **Risperidone**
- **Pimozide**
- **Aripiprazole**

### d. Sleep Related Disorders

Certain movement disorders are also seen among patients with sleep disorders. These are:

- Restless legs syndrome: An irresistible urge to move the legs while at rest, this urge is usually accompanied by an abnormal sensation in the legs, seen only during the evening/night or worsen at this time, relieved by movement and increased by rest. This must be differentiated from akathisia, anxiety, leg myalgia and positional discomfort.

• Periodic limb movement disorder: Brief stereotypic repetitive movements of the legs picked-up during the sleep with the help of polysomnography.

• Sleep-related leg cramps: Nocturnal leg cramps usually the calf and is painful muscle contractions which interfere with the sleep.

• Sleep-related bruxism: Grinding and clenching of teeth during sleep. It can interfere with the sleep of the bed-partner and lead to temporo-mandibular joint dysfunction in the patient. It presents with non-refreshing sleep, temporal headache in the morning and damage to denture.

• Due to substance use/abuse—as a part of withdrawal/ abstinence state: Withdrawal, especially from the hypnotics or alcohol may induce night-terrors, REM sleep behaviour disorder and sleep related myoclonus. Opioid withdrawal is associated with restless legs syndrome.

### Treatment

The treatment of stupor is dependent on its cause. Usually Benzodiazepines are the drugs of choice. The most widely used compound is inj. Lorazepam 2 mg IM or inj. Diazepam 10 mg IV. In addition, ECT (electroconvulsive therapy) is often needed more so among patients with schizophrenia.

Treatment of catatonia/stupor

• **Diagnose the cause**
• **Inj. Lorazepam between 8 and 24 mg/day**
• **ECT**
• **Rule out MNS**
• **Consider alternate medication**

**FURTHER READING**

1. M. Andreasen N, Lopez-Ibor J, Jr. and Geddes JR. New Oxford Textbook of Psychiatry. Gelder Oxford University Press; Oxford: 2009.
2. Ropper, AH, Adams RD, Victor M, Brown RH and Victor M. Adams and Victor's Principles of Neurology. New York; McGraw-Hill Medical Pub. Division: 2005.
3. Sadock B, Sadock VA and Ruiz P. Kaplan and Sadock's Comprehensive Textbook of Psychiatry. Lippincott Williams and Wilkins; Philadeplphia PA: 2009.
4. VanHarten PN, Bakker PR, Mentzel CL, Tijssen MA and Tenback DE. Movement disorders and psychosis, a complex marriage. Front Psychiatry. 2015 Jan 9;5:190.

# 4

# Primary Mental Functions

Jyothsna Chandur, Dharitri Ramaprasad

Mental Status Examination is integral to diagnosis in psychiatry. It is a structured and holistic assessment of the individual's behavioral and cognitive functioning. It includes descriptions of appearance and general behaviour, level of consciousness, motor and speech activity, mood and affect, thought and perception, judgement and insight, and finally the cognitive functions also referred to as primary mental functions. Primary mental functions or cognitive abilities have to do with how a person understands and interacts with the world outside. These are brain-based skills required for carrying out any task from the simplest to the most complex.

A systematic examination of primary mental functions follows a specific order of cortical functions with attention, concentration and memory being the most basic functions on which other higher abilities of language, abstract thinking, reasoning, logical thinking are built. Needless to say that assessment of primary mental functions is an important component to understand the person holistically.

The present chapter attempts to discuss the process of examination of primary mental functions as an important component of Mental Status Examination. The tests commonly used to assess the functions have also been discussed.

Keen observation of the patient's appearance, attitude, and emotional state, verbal and non-verbal behaviour, and style of responding is a pre-requisite for the assessment of primary mental functions as it is for the entire mental status examination and the clinician has to keep these in mind while assessing the performance of the patient on the tests.

37

The assessment of cognitive functions involves a series of well structured, easy-to-administer, standardized, relatively simple set of tests that can be woven into the clinical interview. The principles that are followed in the clinical interview are very important here as well. For example, allowing the patient to feel comfortable, asking questions in a manner that is encouraging and non-threatening to the patient, etc. The presenting symptoms and behavioural observations, during the history-taking, help to generate hypotheses about the nature of the primary disturbance and to plan a strategy for assessment of cognitive functions. A brief evaluation of cognitive functions should enable the clinician to decide whether the patient needs more elaborate assessment. A compilation of all information gathered throughout the interview and MSE leads to the differential diagnosis of the patient. Once the clinician diagnoses the condition, a treatment plan is formulated.

Cognitive functions include all those processes through which an individual perceives, registers, stores, retrieves, and uses information. These tests are hierarchically arranged, with orientation, attention assessed first; followed by memory, new learning and abstract reasoning. Since the basic functions of attention and orientation affect the performance on any other test, such layering of tests helps in interpreting the performance of the patient. For example, if the patient who has severe attention deficits performs poorly on memory and new learning tasks, it would be important for the clinician to analyze the learning deficits keeping in mind the attention deficits exhibited by the patient.

One of the benchmarks to evaluate the performance of the patient on most of these tasks is, approximately 75% accuracy, below which, the performance is considered inadequate. This quantitative measure helps the clinician detect changes in performance over time as well.

## Arousal and Orientation

### Wakefulness/arousal

The level of wakefulness ranges from deep coma to anxious hyper-alertness and is characterized by the intensity of stimulation needed to elicit a meaningful response. In coma or stupor, for example, noxious stimulation is required to provoke a stereotyped response. However, in the normal state of wakefulness, the person is responsive even to the subtlest of cues. Assessment of arousal happens through behavioral observation of the patient. "Comatose," "stuporous," "drowsy," "alert," and "hyper-alert" are terms that are used to describe the level of arousal.

Most psychiatric patients are either alert and awake or in a few cases somnolent or lethargic. Delirious, stuporous and comatose patients are not as common in the field of psychiatry as in neurology and neurosurgery.

Needless to elaborate, the level of arousal of the person significantly impacts the performance on any of the tests. Testing of attention and concentration is feasible only in patients whose awareness or consciousness is not grossly disturbed. Observational and investigative methods change when one examines patients with disturbance in the levels of awareness.

## Orientation

The process by which an individual 'grasps' his/her environment and locates himself/herself in relation to it is known as orientation. There are four aspects to orientation: person, place, time and situation. If a person 'gets'his position in reference to time; appreciates his/her situation as to both space and circumstances; and understands his/her relationship to other individuals, s/he is said to be oriented. The following questions help establish the orientation of the individual with regard to all the four aspects. They need to be carefully framed in order to maintain the non-threatening attitude, yet, establishing the seriousness.

## Sample Questions

1. What is your name?
2. What day is it today? What is the date today?
3. Can you tell me what time it could be now?
4. Do you know where you have come?
5. Could you tell me why you have come here (have been brought here)?
6. Why are we having this examination?

Most of the times, it is helpful to weave in these questions as part of the initial interview, i.e. as a part of the introductions. If there is anything significant, then a slightly more formal set of questions, deliberately asked would be of help. There is no hard and fast rule about the order in which these questions need to be asked. The clinician will have to use his/her judgement regarding the exact framing and the order of the questions.

Orientation to time and situation are more easily disturbed as compared to the other two aspects, especially in the acute phase of psychiatric disorders, or illnesses like delirium. However, very intense emotional reactions may also lead to disorientation at times. Later stages of dementia can bring about more serious problems in all the four aspects. If there is disorientation, more often than not, there will be disturbances in the other cognitive functions as well.

## Attention

The testing of attention is a more refined consideration of the state of wakefulness than the level of arousal. Attention is the conscious, selective process by which the organism scans the sensory inputs obtained from the internal and the external world to select those that should be given priority. It is a selective process and hence, involves vigilance. From among the several sensory stimuli that make their impact on the organism at any point in time, a few are scanned and selected for further processing.

Along with the interpretation of the patient's performance on the tests, it is important to observe the behaviour of the patient which can yield specific clues about the underlying deficits. Reaction times are usually longer in patients who have deficits in attention. This is most often evident even in the initial phase of the clinical interview and suggests to the examiner a possibility of attention deficit.

· Some individuals become highly distracted with the subjective internal stimuli from their internal world. This makes it impossible for them to 'attend' to the objective external world. It is difficult to elicit the attention of such individuals who are 'preoccupied'. The narrowing down of interest on to one part of the sensory inputs that are attended to and maintaining it over a period of time is known as concentration. It is clear that concentration implies a certain amount of tenacity and persistence over a period of time. The inability to hold the attention over a sufficient period of time because of the interference of the fleeting stimuli which seem to redirect the attention of the individual who is lacking in tenacity, is known as distractibility. A clinician is interested in knowing whether a patient can demonstrate purposeful attention, is too distractible, unable to maintain concentration or is preoccupied.

An ideal test for attention should try to assess focus on a simple task, while placing minimal demand on other functions like language, motor activity and so on. This would tease out the pure attention deficits from the deficits in sensory or other cognitive functions. However, this is easier said than done, since almost all the tasks involve multiple functions at the same time.

**Some of the commonly used tests are given below:**

1. **Digit Span Test:** The examiner verbally presents a series of digits, taking care to present them slowly, distinctly, without grouping them. Then, the patient is asked to repeat the digit series.

   Later, the examiner presents a new series of digits and asks the patient to repeat them in the reverse order, i.e. the digit given at the end by the examiner is to be repeated first by the patient and then the previous one and so on. Thus the complete series is recalled in the reverse order. In both these series, the examiner starts with 3 digits and gradually increases up to 9. Ability to repeat 6/7 digits forward and 4/5 digits backward is considered adequate for an average Indian adult. Generally the difference between the digit forwards and backwards is not greater than 2 digits.

   Following series of digits can be used:

| Digit Forward | Digit Backward |
|---|---|
| 3 – 8 | 2 – 7 |
| 5 – 9 – 2 | 1 – 8 – 6 |
| 4 – 8 – 3 – 7 | 3 – 7 – 2 – 5 |
| 3 – 1 – 4 – 6 – 9 | 9 – 3 – 4 – 8 – 6 |
| 9 – 3 – 5 – 8 – 4 – 2 | 4 – 2 – 8 – 6 – 1 – 3 |
| 6 – 9 – 3 – 1 – 7 – 5 – 2 | 2 – 1 – 7 – 3 – 5 – 9 – 4 |

The same test, digit span is also used to assess the immediate recall and the working memory.

2. **Serial Subtraction:** The patient is asked to subtract 7 from 100 serially until the remainder is less than 7. Alternative tests: Subtract 3 from 40 or count backwards from 20 to 1 (both are easier as compared to the first alternative).

   The performance can be accepted as normal if the time taken is less than 2 minutes and the patient has not committed more than 2 errors.

3. Another test is to read out a string of letters to the patient in which one letter is repeated frequently. The patient is asked to tap on the table each time the repeated letter is heard. For example, "Please tap each time you hear the letter M."M L M B K M N Z K M M K G M H W M L T M ...

4. **Digit Vigilance:** The patient is given a sheet filled with random numbers or alphabets. He/she is asked to mark/ cancel a particular number or alphabet starting from the first row all the way to the end of the sheet. Anything more than 7–8 minutes is considered to be inadequate. This test is not conducted routinely as a part of the MSE. However, if the clinician detects a deficit in attention, digit vigilance test would help the clinician decide whether an elaborate neuropsychological assessment would benefit the patient.

The pattern of sustained concentration in performance is more informative than the accuracy of the responses. It is important to note whether the patient performed these simple functions on the test within an appropriate time span or if his reactions were too slow. If the latter is true, the time interval between the question and the response should be noted. Disturbances in attention are reflected in the person's inability to persist at a task, perseveration, distractibility or an inability to control immediate and inappropriate responses.

Attention and concentration are affected by many different factors such as interest, motivation, intense emotions and physical factors like hunger, fatigue and so on. Attention and concentration are also affected in psychiatric illnesses like schizophrenia, depression, anxiety. Severe disturbances are seen in lesions and other neurological illnesses as well.

**Memory and New Learning**

Memory is the function through which information acquired through attention and observation is stored and retained to be brought back to conscious awareness when necessary. Memory of an individual is modified on the basis of his/ her emotional needs. For the purpose of description, memory may be considered as consisting of three processes:

The act of committing something to memory, i.e.'encoding' (input); holding the material in memory, i.e. 'storage'; and remembering (recalling) that material, i.e. 'retrieval' (output).

Forgetting is the process by which previously acquired information is lost because of the lapse of time, disuse, or as a result of the continuous organizing process of memory.

Memory deficit, whatever the cause, is referred to as amnesia, and it can result from brain damage, disease or injury. There may be a selective or generalized loss of memory, which can be temporary or permanent, and the deficit may affect short-term storage, long-term storage or both.

Anterograde amnesia is the inability to form new memories and learn new information.

Retrograde amnesia refers to the inability to recall information stored/occurring before the injury. However, the ability to learn new information remains unaffected.

Assessment of memory involves integrating both the information given by the patient and the informant (during the interview and history taking) as well as the formal yet brief assessment using the following tests.

**Immediate recall** (less than 10/15 seconds) can be viewed as synonymous with the ability to attend and is not strictly speaking, a function of retention.

- Digit span forward measures immediate recall. Digit span backward, requires mental processing and measures working memory as well.

**Short-term memory:** Information is processed and stored for a short period of time and retrieved when necessary, in other words, ability to register and retain.

This can be assessed by asking the patient to recall and describe some events of the past 24 hours and confirming the accuracy of the responses from the informants. Questions like the following may be asked:

- When did you come to the hospital?
- With whom did you come?
- How did you come here?
- What did you eat for breakfast/lunch?
- Whom did you meet today?

In addition following tests help to assess short-term memory:

- The patient is asked to learn four unrelated objects or concepts, a short sentence, or a five-component name and address, and asked to recall the information in 3 to 5 minutes after performing a second, unrelated cognitive task.
- Drilled word span test: (This is not a part of the routine MSE. However, it is conducted when the clinician wants to gather more information regarding the patient's memory)

  1. A list of words which are unrelated to one another (usually equal to the patient's forward digit span minus one) are read out clearly and slowly to the patient. The list is read repeatedly until the entire list is recalled by the patient for three consecutive times. This is referred to as the criterion.

  2. After this the patient is instructed to remain silent for sixty seconds.At the end of sixty seconds, the patient is asked to repeat the entire list. If he is not able to, then this may signify that the patient is internally distracted or lacks initiative, and the list is presented again until 'the criterion'is reached, that is, the patient recalls the entire list three consecutive times.

  3. Recall is then tested after another interval of 60 seconds, during which the patient is distracted with some other mental activity. For example, serial subtraction.

  4. If the list is not recalled in its entirety after 60 seconds or 3 minutes, recognition can be tested by reading out a list of words which includes the original list as well as distractors and asking the patient to indicate the words that occurred in the original list.

The number of times the list needs to be presented to reach criterion (for immediate recall and also after the 60-second silent interval) is a measure of problems in attention. The effect of distraction is determined by comparing the number of words recalled following the silent and the distracted 60-second recall trials. Patients who have amnesia but no attention deficits can rehearse and remember information for a specific period of time if not distracted but lose the information once distracted, suggestive of deficits in encoding. The rate of forgetting over time can be measured by comparing the number of words recalled after 1 minute and 3 minute intervals with distraction.

**Long-term memory or remote memory** can be tested by the patient's ability to recall remote personal (e.g. when was your son born? When did you finish high school?) or historic events (e.g. when did India attain independence? Who was the first prime minister of Independent India?). These specific questions asked should pertain to information that has occurred more than 8–10 years ago. Obviously, in asking remote personal events, the clinician must be privy to accurate information to judge the accuracy of the patient's response or should later check with the family members to test the accuracy of information. If the patient is able to give a chronological account of his/her life, then this is suggestive of a reasonably good long term memory.

**Working memory** refers to processes of brief on-line holding and manipulation of information. This is a cognitive function, that is, most often affected in patients with psychotic illnesses like schizophrenia.

1. Digit span—especially backwards, measures working memory

2. Letter-number sequencing (subtest of the Wechsler Memory Scale-III) is also used for this purpose. A string of letters intermixed with numbers (e.g. J w 6 h 3 a 2) is presented aloud. The patient must repeat the stimuli in ascending order, with numbers first (in ascending order) followed by the alphabets in the alphabetical order (i.e. 2 3 6 a h j w).

An oft reported side effect of ECT is memory impairment. In most cases, this resembles the amnesic pattern where there is loss of memory for events following the administration of ECT (anterograde amnesia), and sometimes some retrograde amnesia too, so that the person may not recall the events leading up to the treatment. There is invariably improvement over time, and often, a brief retrograde amnesia (of a day or two) is all that remains. Before interpreting the performance one needs to make sure if the patient has undergone ECT in case he/she is already under treatment.

## Intelligence

Intelligence refers to the ability to think abstractly and adapt to new situations. It is more formally described by Wechsler as 'the global capacity to think rationally, act purposefully and deal effectively with the environment'.

In the context of Mental Status Examination, we evaluate the intelligence of a person quickly, usually to get an overall view rather than a detailed profile.

Intelligence is a general ability and colours every test performance. During the mental status examination, the individual's performance varies depending on the intellectual ability. It is known that the complexity and the content of the symptomatology is also dependent to a certain extent on the intellectual level of the patient. A clinician therefore assesses the intelligence of the patient clinically during the very first mental status examination though he may later follow it up with a psychological referral if and when necessary. By evaluating vocabulary, abstraction and general information, the clinician can have a general idea of the patient's intelligence.

## Vocabulary

The size and the clarity of the patient's vocabulary is often a useful measure to gauge the individual's intellectual functioning. The patient is asked to define different words of differing degrees of difficulty and complexity ranging from concrete concepts referring to objects to concepts that are abstract. For example, ball, chair, law, pity, shame.

## Abstraction Capacity

The ability of the individual to reason and use abstract concepts are measured using the following tests:

- Similarities and Differences: The clinician presents two words to the individual who is asked to identify the differences between the two. For example, mosquito and a fly; tv and radio. A slightly more difficult test is to identity the similarities between two words. For example, orange and apple; iron and silver.
- Proverbs: The individual is presented with a proverb and asked to explain its meaning. For example, "Barking dogs seldom bite".

In both the tests measuring abstraction, the clinician pays attention to whether the patient is able to move beyond the concrete level to the abstract level.

### General Information

In eliciting the range and depth of general information possessed by the patient, the questions have to be chosen with regard to the patient's background.

Some of the questions that can be asked:

- What are the colours in our National flag?
- Name any five vegetables or flowers.
- At what time of the day is the person's shadow the shortest?
- Name any five rivers in India.
- What metal is attracted by magnets?
- Why does the moon look larger than the sun?
- If your shadow is pointing towards northeast while you stand, where is the sun?

While making an impression about the intelligence of the individual with the help of the performance on vocabulary, abstraction and general information, one should keep in mind, the education level (highest grade passed), vocation (whether currently working or previous vocation), socio-economic status and the functioning level of the individual before he/she developed the illness.

There are times when the clinician notices that the intellectual functioning as seen currently during the MSE may be lower than what the previous record suggests or what the relatives or the patient himself describes. This deterioration in the intellectual functioning could be due to the damage caused by the illness. In such cases a detailed evaluation is warranted.

Intelligence is more accurately assessed using standardized psychological tests like the Progressive Matrices, Wechsler's scales, Bhatia's battery of tests. These psychometrically sound assessments give a detailed profile of the individual's intelligence including a quantified measure of intelligence, called the Intelligence Quotient (IQ). An IQ within the range of 90 – 110 is considered average. Below 90, it is considered to be decreasing with an IQ of 70 being the cut off. An individual with an IQ score of 70 and below is considered to have mental retardation. On the other hand, IQ levels beyond 110 are considered to be above average, superior and so on.

## Motivation and Mood

Level of motivation of the patient is one of the important factor to be considered while assessing cognitive functions. The clinician needs to observe as to how motivated the patient is during the assessment since this also can have a significant impact on the performance on all the tests. Some of the obvious ways that can be observed are, the patient's co-operation, sustained effort, show of initiative during the assessment. Patients who are not motivated may respond with an "I don't know" very frequently.

Depression would be one of the psychiatric conditions where the motivation and the interest of the patient would be very low. In illnesses like anxiety, the motivation to take the tests could be affected because of the agitation and preoccupation. Very low motivation would be very common in neurological conditions as well.

Since the clinician would have made enough observations regarding the patient's mood during the course of the interview, he would have to carefully separate the mood related disturbances from the underlying cognitive disturbances in order to reach accurate diagnosis and treatment plan.

## Cognitive functions are assessed during the following situations

1. When the clinician is meeting the individual for the first time as a part of case history interview and mental status examination (during the initial interview).
2. On admission to and discharge from an institution.

3. Before making important health care decisions especially the ones which are related to the individual's capacity.
4. Following major changes in medication.
5. The individual's behaviour that is unusual for him/her and/or inappropriate to the situation.

## Cautions while assessing cognitive functions

1. Interpretation of the tests should be holistically done, considering all aspects of the assessment. The observations about behaviour of the patient throughout the interview, the attitude, interest, mood, comprehension all aid in the interpretation of the performance.

2. The clinician needs to conduct the assessment as far as possible in the language that the patient is most comfortable with, since comprehension of instructions and/or ease of response will have a very significant impact on performance on all the tests. If this is not possible for some reason, it is important to document the language in which the assessment was conducted so as to help in the interpretation. It is important for the clinician to ensure that the patient has understood the instructions clearly before conducting any of the tests. Some ways of ensuring this are, to ask the patient to repeat the instructions or wherever possible, conduct a trial round before the actual test.

3. It is important to record the responses of the patient verbatim clearly (along with date and time usually) while conducting the assessment. Such clear documentation will not only ensure accurate diagnosis, it will also help to chart the progress of the patient over time.

## Other tests to assess cognitive functions

Some of the other tests which are standardized and can be administered quickly in order to screen the cognitive functions of patients are listed below. However, almost all of these are used in neruo-degenerative conditions like dementia.

- Mental Status Questionnaire (Kahn and Goldfarb, 1960):10 questions, selected from 31 in the original instrument that had the greatest discriminating power for "organicity."
- The Mini-Mental Status Examination (Folstein et al., 1975): Perhaps the most widely used "short, portable" mental status

test. This is a 30-point test with 10 points devoted to orientation, 3 to registration, 5 to calculation, 3 to short-term memory, 8 to language function, and 1 to constructional ability.

• The Neurobehavioral Cognitive Status Examination (Kieran, Mueller, Langston and Van Dyke, 1987): A screening examination that assesses cognition in a brief but quantitative fashion, uses independent tests to evaluate functioning within five major cognitive ability areas: Language, constructions, memory, calculations, and reasoning. The examination separately assesses level of consciousness, orientation, and attention.

• Short Portable Mental Status Questionnaire (Pfeiffer, 1975): A 10 item questionnairze that helps screen elderly patients with dementia or other neuro-degenerative conditions.

Assessment of cognitive functions involves a dynamic exploration of cognitive, behavioural, and emotional abnormalities resulting from a psychiatric/neurological dysfunction. An accurate history and a complete MSE are the crucial first steps in the assessment and are the only diagnostic tools clinicians have to select and plan the treatment for any patient. So, an assessment based on these considerations should provide a summary of the deficits, their effects on test performance, their impact on daily living, and their implications for diagnosis and management of the illness.

## FURTHER READING

1. Cowen, P., Harrisson, P. and Burns, T. (2012). Shorter Oxford Textbook of Psychiatry (6th ed). Oxford University Press, UK.

2. Kaplan, HI and Sadock, B. J. (1999). Concise Textbook of Clinical Psychiatry (7th ed). Williams and Williams, Baltimore.

3. Kay, J., and Tasman, A. (2006). Essentials of Psychiatry, John Wiley and Sons, Ltd, Chichester, UK.

4. Kolb, B., Whishaw, I.Q. (2007). Fundamentals of human neuropsychology (6th ed). New York, NY: Worth Publishers.

5. Mesulam, M. M. (2000). Principles of cognitive and behavioral neurology, (2nd ed). Oxford University Press, New York, 174–256.

6. Prabhu, GG (1999). Primary Mental Functions, in Namboodri, VMD, John, CJ and Subbalakshmi, TP. (Eds). Clinical methods in Psychiatry, (2nd ed). New Delhi: B. I. Churchill Livingston, 42–54.
7. Puri, BK and Treasaden (2011). Textbook of Psychiatry (3rd ed). Elsevier.

# 5

# Anomalies of Perception

VMD Namboodiri

Perception may be defined as that process by which data from the sense organs are meaningfully organised and interpreted in the light of past experience. It is both an active and complex process. Active, because it involves organisation and synthesis of sensory stimuli and these are active, not static, phenomena. Complex, because it incorporates multiple independent processes occurring simultaneously as sensation, association and interpretation. Incoming sensory data obtained through the receptor organs such as the eye, ear, etc. are linked with past knowledge somewhere in the association areas of the brain, resulting in meaningful interpretation of the new stimuli. This is perception through which we understand objects in their appropriate identity, as sun, trees, house or man.

## SENSATION AND PERCEPTION

Differentiation is to be made between sensation and perception. Sensations are the end result of stimulations of the sensory organs and *per se* are not meaningful. It is only one step in the complex process of perception. To make it meaningful many data available at a particular point of time in the sensory field may have to be eliminated and only the relevant ones retained. These are combined with similar relevant data from other sensory fields which altogether make a sensory percept experienced as a "sensory configuration" which again are without recognition. These are analysed and interpreted in the light of past knowledge in the association areas as mentioned above which leads to meaningful recognition of the object or data.

## SENSATION AND IMAGERY

Perceptions are mixed with imagery (fantasy) in our "stream of consciousness" and are experienced as a composite whole. But a person has no difficulty in chaffing out one from the other, the "real" from the "imagined" one. Perception occurs in the external space ("out there"), whereas the images in fantasy occur in the internal space ("in here"). fantasies are created voluntarily and are volitional. Memories and fantasies pervade a person's mental activity along with normal perceptions. Daydreaming involves perceptions from different sense modalities and from different times admixed with fantasy. People vary considerably in their ability to do this.

Obviously perception is extremely important in day-to-day life. Knowledge of the identity of an object and its apparent stability gives a feeling of security and directs us to react 'accordingly to the object or situation. Damaging accidents occur when actions are guided by erroneous perceptions, as in automobile traffic conditions when the red light is perceived as green or in social situations where somebody's anger is mistaken for joy.

## SELECTIVITY OF PERCEPTION

It would seem natural to think that a set of stimuli give rise to the same percepts (units of perception) always. That is, the same stimuli convey the same percepts at all times and to all people. This is not so. Perceptions are highly selective. They are coloured by the individual's set, values, learning, interest mood, fantasies and many other factors. As an example may be quoted the Chinese letters which to an outsider are only meaningless chaos of lines. In the famous hovel of Nathaniel Hawthorne, "The Scarlet Letter" the letter "A" had a special meaning to its characters, which branded Hester Pryss as an adulteress.

All sense organs contribute to the formation of percepts. Perception is impaired in sensory deficits like blindness and deafness, but not lost because cues from other sensory channels are still operational.

## Types of Perception

Individual sense organs provide data for perceptions related to the respective sensory modality as auditory, visual, tactile, etc. But there are many special types of perceptions which are wholly an inter-sensory affair, as time and movement. There are no special space and time senses and the sensory cues intervening between two points of time or distance give hints for appreciating them. Perception of movement involves space and time simultaneously. It is proposed that psychological appreciation of time is functionally connected to the individual's body functions, i.e. to the circadian rhythms (e.g. respiration, pulse, etc.) and rate of physiological processes in general, which furnish cues about the lapse of time.

## Apperception

Apperception is recognition of what the perceptual data means. It is the ability to understand perceptions in their proper context. In the face of clear perception an incorrect interpretation means faulty apperception. Agnosias are in fact disturbances of apperception. When the subject matter becomes difficult, apperception becomes delayed. Other factors affecting apperception are the level of intelligence, disturbances in retention (e.g. Korsakoff's syndrome) and altered sensorium of the perceiver. (e.g. delirium). Apperception is grossly disturbed when registration is impaired or lost as in alcohol blackouts. The heavy drinker while continuing drinking acts and behaves "normally" but is unable to recall at a later stage the events which occurred during the "black out period".

## ANOMALIES OF PERCEPTION

These can be considered under the following four heads:

1. Sensory distortions

2. Sensory deceptions

3. Perceptual disturbances of time and space

4. Perceptual disturbances of awareness of the body

## 1. Sensory Distortions

Sensory distortion may occur in any sensory modality. Here the object is real but its sensory attributes are altered. Mainly they are of two types: (a) changes in intensity and (b) changes in quality.

### Changes in Intensity

The sensations become more intense and more vivid (hyperesthesia) or vice versa (hypoesthesia). In the former sounds are heard louder and colours appear brighter. A pinprick produces excruciating pain. In hypoesthesia the sensations are dull and diminished and pain may be reduced (hypalgia) or absent (analgia).

In both hypo-aesthesia and hyper-aesthesia there is no deterioration or improvement in the functioning of the sensory organs or their perceptions. It is only a mere change in their threshold-lower in hyper-aesthesia and higher in hypo-aesthesia. In hyperacusis even normal conversation or whispering at a long distance is perceived abnormally intense or loud.

Hyperesthesia occurs under intense emotions where the psychological threshold is lowered. This is seen in acute psychosis and prior to epileptic seizures. In delirium, on the other hand, the threshold is raised and hypoesthesia particularly with regard to auditory stimuli occurs (hypoacusis). Hypalgesia and analgesia may be neurological in origin or sometimes present as a dissociative symptom or under hypnosis.

### Changes in Quality

Some drugs and toxic substances when consumed are liable to produce these changes (e.g. yellow vision or xanthopia with Santonin; or metallic taste in the mouth with Metronidazole). In micropsia objects are seen smaller than their normal size and farther away (as looking from the other end of a telescope) and in macropsia they are larger and closer. In dysmegalopsia they are larger on one side and smaller on the other. They occur in organic conditions, e.g. parieto-temporal lobe lesions, epilepsy and sometimes in schizophrenia. Sometimes one quality shifts to another as occurs under the effect of psychedelic drugs where infinite hues of colour are perceived by the user.

## 2. Sensory Deceptions

The two main sensory deceptions are illusions and hallucinations.

### a. Illusions

Sensory deceptions are differentiated from sensory distortions in that in the former there is an altogether new set of perceptions which occur in the presence or absence of an external stimulus. If the external stimulus is present, it is called an illusion, if not, a hallucination.

To illustrate: Suppose a piece of rope is perceived as a rope which however assumes a colour different from its original one. This is sensory distortion. If it is perceived as a snake, probably because of the fading light, it is an illusion, but if the observer 'sees' a rope or a snake where there is none, it is called a hallucination.

### Causes of Illusions

a. Inadequate sensory input: This occurs when the person is inattentive or when the environment fails to provide enough cues (e.g. darkness).
b. Affect: Walking in the wood at night in a state of anxiety and loneliness, a tree trunk is mistaken for a lurking animal.
c. Set and needs: Subjects who are hungry or starving often perceive food and eatables concealed in an ambiguous drawing.
d. Imagery: Ill-defined markings as in clouds or blotches on the wall give rise to meaningful forms to some individuals without any conscious effort on their part (pareidolia).

### Clinical Significance

Illusions do not necessarily imply psychopathology and can occur even in normal people particularly when the surroundings are not clear enough (e.g. semidarkness, noisy room) or when the person labours under stress (apprehension and fear). In illness states they are common in delirium, intoxication with drugs and severe emaciation.

Perceptions which disagree with physical stimuli are also termed illusions. A spoon immersed in a glass of water appears bent. The figures 3 and 8, and the letters B and. K appear to have two equal halves. This is a physical illusion. Turn the book upside down and see that their upper and lower halves are unequal. Muller-Lyer illusion is another example. These have no clinical significance.

Illusions should be distinguished from misinterpretations. Misinterpretations are wrong deductions happening at a thinking level. An example is misinterpreting a piece of yellow metal for a gold coin. The differentiating features are: (a) the perceptions are unaltered and (b) it is easily reversible even if the perceptual field is unaltered.

Illusions are to be distinguished from functional hallucinations also (see below). Both occur in response to an external stimulus. In functional hallucinations however both the external stimulus and the new percept occur simultaneously, whereas in illusions the provoking stimulus is incorporated in the new percept and is not therefore perceived separately.

### b. Hallucinations

Hallucinations are false perceptions which occur in the "absence" of corresponding sensory stimuli. Subjectively they are indistinguishable of normal perceptions. What the doctor calls a hallucination, is a "normal sensory experience to the patient". The only cues to the patient that it could be a hallucination are: (1) Physical impossibility of its occurrence and (2) that others are not sharing his experience. Hallucinations occur along with normal perceptions. Cultural factors greatly modify the content of hallucinations as well as how the patient describes them.

The above description is deficient as it does not cover functional hallucinations (because in functional hallucinations there is an external stimulus) while it erroneously includes dream states which are not true hallucinations. To avoid this, Jaspers defined hallucinations as false perceptions which are not sensory distortions and which occur along with real perceptions simultaneously.

## Classification

**Depending on the sense of modality.** Hallucinations occur in all modalities of sensation and are named accordingly.

**Auditory.** Noises, musical tones, accusatory voices.

**Visual.** Flashes of light, visual patterns, animals, people.

**Olfactory.** Smells which are agreeable or not.

**Gustatory.** Pertaining to the sense of taste. Altered taste of food which patient might attribute to mixing of poison.

**Tactile.** They are either light or deep. In the former, patient reports of being touched, often stroked or tickled, he reports of insects or worms crawling over his body or just under the skin. In the latter, patient reports of muscle being twisted or torn or says his internal organs are being crushed.

**Vestibular.** Flying through air or nose-diving from great heights.

**Sense of 'presence'.** Some people often get a strange perception that they are being followed or that somebody is beside them, even though they are alone. This can occur as a hallucinatory experience.

**Formed and unformed.** Perceptions may be elementary or unformed like sparks and flashes of light. Sometimes they are partly organised as sounds and visual patterns. Often hallucinations are formed and meaningful as vision of people and objects, voices talking each other, etc.

**Simple and complex.** In simple hallucinations, only one sensory modality is involved (as vision or hearing). In complex, multiple modalities are involved at the same time, as a wildfire, where visual (tongues of flame), auditory (crackling wood) and olfactory (fumes of smoke) perceptions occur simultaneously.

**True and false.** True hallucinations have reality value to the patient and they urge him to act according to their content. This is absent in pseudo-hallucinations in which patient recognises that his perceptions are hot real and that they have no basis.

## Special types of Hallucinations

**Hypnagogic and hypnopompic hallucinations.** Hypnagogic hallucinations are those which occur in drowsy state prior to falling sleep. Hypnopompic hallucinations are those which emerge while waking up from a deep sleep, again in the drowsy state. They are usually visual but may include voices, often indistinct. Sometimes the subject hears his own name being called.

**Functional hallucinations.** In functional hallucinations there is a provoking stimulus which is experienced along with the hallucination. The bird chirrups and the patient hears God talking to him: He hears people deriding him when the radio is switched on. The radio music and the sinister remarks of people are both heard at the same time.

**Synaesthesiae (reflex hallucination).** Frequently stimulation in one sensory field produces sensations pertaining to another and both are perceived simultaneously by the patient. This is synaesthesia. For example, with every sound heard one patient experienced a painful tap on her head. A provoking visual hallucination is another example.

**Extracampine hallucinations.** Hallucinations experienced outside the limits of the respective sensory fields are termed extracampine. For example, seeing through the back of one's head, hearing voices of people talking many kilometres away.

**Scenic (panoramic) hallucinations.** Vivid, continuous and complex hallucinations of an event depicting even the minutest detail.

**Somatic hallucinations.** These are hallucinatory experiences of the whole body or parts of the body. Phantom limb and autoscopy are examples, (see below). Sexual hallucinations (erection, orgasm, penetration) are other examples of somatic hallucinations.

Hallucinations vary in their clarity of perception, richness of details and duration. Hallucinations of several sense modalities can occur concurrently. Hallucinations can also occur along with illusions posing difficulty in distinguishing them.

Depending on the content of hallucinations the accompanying affect also differs (joy, anger, anxiety, grief).

## Causes of Hallucinations

**Drugs.** There are many drugs which when used even in pharmacological doses produce abnormalities of perception without grossly altering consciousness. These are called psychotomimetic drugs, also known as hallucinogens or psychedelic drugs. The most common among these are LSD, Mescaline, Amphetamines and Cannabis.

**Sensory deprivation.** Persons subjected to prolonged isolation (e.g. shipwrecked sailors, polar explorers, prisoners in solitary confinement) have hallucinatory experiences. The same phenomena are noted when a normal individual is artificially deprived of his sensory inputs when characteristic symptoms like anxiety, distractibility and perceptual disturbances appear within a period ranging from a few hours to a few days. Deprivation of auditory, visual and tactile stimuli are the most crucial. Patients who gradually lose vision secondary to an eye disease sometimes report visual hallucinations.

**Emotions.** In depression with guilt and self reproach the patient experiences hallucinations upbraiding him.

**Hypnosis and trance states.** Here hallucinations are induced by powerful suggestion. These disappear when the subject comes out of the state.

**Disorders of CNS.** Lesions of cortex produce hallucinations, nature of which depends on the site of lesion (visual cortex— visual hallucinations). In epilepsy, hallucinations of all sensory modalities are seen.

**Other conditions.** Hallucinations are seen in a host of other conditions also, like starvation, sleep deprivation, febrile illness, deficiency states and metabolic illness.

## Conditions Simulating Hallucinations

**After images.** After images are either positive or negative. Looking at a bright light (or sun) or colours for sometime, when the gaze is diverted to a gray wall, the original bright image or the colour is seen to persist for some .time. This is the positive after image—positive because it is similar in hue and brightness. Often it gives way to a negative after image which is opposite in brightness or hue to the original. This is familiar to those who watch the TV news. A negative after image of the reader persists on the screen for a few seconds when TV is switched off. After images occur in movement also. After looking at a water fall, to some, if the eyes, are turned to the bank the trees appear to swim upward.

**Eidetic images**. These are also known as photographic images, and sensory phenomena where the individual is able to retain the image of an original stimulus (visual or auditory) in all clarity, details and vividness even after the stimulus is removed. They are not often images as these can be recalled after a long time, are not complementary and are not exact copies of the original stimulus.

**Memory images.** These should be differentiated from hallucinations. Differentiating features are:

| Hallucinations | Memory images |
|---|---|
| a. Occur in the external objective space. Has an 'out there' feeling | Occur in the internal objective space (in the 'mind's eye' or 'ear') |
| b. Are clearly defined and complete | Are not clearly defined. Are incomplete, only individual details are prominent |
| c. Has concrete reality | Patient recognizes them as the product of their imagination and having no factual basis. |
| d. Remain constant, and unchanged | Fade off but can be recreated at will. |
| e. Occur independent of the will | Are under the control of the will (voluntary). |

### Examination of a Hallucinating Patient

Overt behaviour of a patient often gives clues that he is hallucinating. The patient sits gazing into space fixedly and constantly or to a particular point attentively for long periods of time. During conversation his eyes are seen tracking a moving object in space or return to a particular place again and again. Fleety eye movements as if to catch the source of a sound which he 'hears' is another clue. Wearing a countenance of listening to 'voices from the sky', lip movements suggesting that he is muttering or conversing with a third person are all behavioural cues which implicate that the patient is hallucinating.

Many a time the patient might voluntarily report to the doctor of his strange experiences. Patients differ in their way of descriptions. For example, in auditory hallucinations the patients may deny of hearing voices speaking to him but instead says that spoken messages are transferred to his mind which he can hear (differentiate from "thought insertion", see below). Sometimes he would withhold any information even they have been referred to earlier deny them when confronted by the doctor, in such cases the doctor must continue his efforts to overcome the patient's fear or resistance in reporting his experiences and try to elicit these vital signs.

When evidence favours assumption that the patient is frankly hallucinating he can be directly asked about his experiences "Have you at anytime heard your name being called, even though you are sure you were alone?" "Did you ever have strange experiences like your thoughts being answered back or read aloud?" "Do unseen people talk bad things about you or tell what you should do?". "Do they keep on telling things which you are doing?" Questions similar to above might elicit fruitful responses. Questions should be tailored to cover other sense modalities also—like "Do you often get strange sensations on your skin—as if a worm is crawling, though you can't see any" "Do you get strange and unusual tastes in your mouth?" Once the patient confirms them by answering positively the examiner should try to get more information about his hallucinations. In the auditory modality he may be asked "Could you identify the voice?" "How many voices were talking to you?" "Was it a male voice or a female voice?" "Was it friendly or threatening?" "What other things do the voices tell you?" "Why do you think they are telling these to you?"

In milder forms where the patient is guarded or denies his experiences, queries should be non-direct and more subtle though in these cases also the examiner should attempt to gather as much information as possible regarding the hallucinatory experience.

In evaluating the hallucinations or any other perceptual disturbances, the following points also should be considered.

1. Sensory modality involved: Auditory, visual, tactile. Are more than one modalities involved and which ones?

2. Nature of perception: Whether the perceptions are 'out there' in the space or 'in the mind'. Their intensity, clarity, frequency. Do the voices give a running commentary?

3. Can they be initiated voluntarily? Or stopped at will by the patient?

4. Circumstances eliciting the experience: Time of the day, in waking state or while drowsy? Medication? Physical state and associated illness, if any.

5. Insight and reality value: Does the patient believe that the experiences are factual? Or does he think that they are products of his imagination?

6. Content of the hallucinations: Personal comments? Commands? Accusatory? Threatening?

7. Attitude of the patient to the hallucinations; associated effect—pleasing or disturbing?

8. Reaction of patient to the hallucinations: Unbothered? Does he try to avoid them by closing the ears or eyes? Does he obey the commands? Does he reply or converse with the 'voices'? Does he attempt to escape from the scene?

9. Are there associated perceptual disturbances also as illusions, disturbances related to time, space and patient's body image and self (see below)?

10. Are there associated sensory distortions also as described in the beginning of the chapter?

### Clinical Significance

Hallucinations almost always are hallmarks of psychosis though they at times occur in some non-psychotic conditions. The hypnagogic and hypnopompic hallucinations occur in normal people also. All types of hallucinations can occur in all types of psychosis. Hallucinations are non-specific and do not help in differential diagnosis of the illness. However, the following account obeys the conventional description of hallucinations in relation to their clinical significance.

Hallucinations of all modalities occur in schizophrenia but auditory hallucinations are the commonest. Auditory hallucinations occurring in a clear consciousness are strongly suggestive of schizophrenia, though these can be seen in other psychoses as well. Somatic hallucinations including sexual ones (erection and orgasm) and tactile hallucinations (insects crawling under the skin; animal inside the body) and kinaesthetic hallucinations occur frequently in schizophrenia. If there are visual hallucinations; they are usually accompanied by hallucinatory experiences in other sensory modalities also.

Some types of auditory hallucinations have been described. as characteristic of schizophrenia: (a) thought echo (*'echo de la pense'*) where patient hears his own thought read aloud, (b) hearing hallucinatory voices arguing each other, often referring to the patient in the third person and (c) voices that give a running commentary on the patient's activities.

In mania, hallucinations are rare. If present, they are usually auditory. In depression, auditory hallucinations may occur reproaching the patient and asking him to kill himself. Unlike in schizophrenia where the hallucinations occur throughout the day, in depression hallucination have a diurnal variation and occur more frequently when the patient is alone.

Hallucinations induced by psychedelic drugs are more commonly visual and occasionally auditory—perceptions of other senses also occur at times. Infrequently there are a melée of senses and synaesthesiae which the subjects fantastically describe as 'hearing the colour', 'seeing the sounds'. The hallucinations are often colourful mosaics and geometrical patterns.

In dissociative states and in temporal lobe epilepsy, scenic (panoramic) hallucinations are commonly recounted. In the former they might relate to a past event having some emotional significance to the patient.

All modalities of sensations can be involved in epilepsy. Visual (occipital discharges), auditory (temporal discharges) and olfactory (uncal discharges) are the most common. In psychic seizures (temporal lobe attacks) the hallucinations are complex, vivid and three dimensional. *deja vu* and *jamais vu* experiences occasionally accompany the fits.

Visual hallucinations of a frightening nature are usually seen in delirium where illusions intermingle with hallucinations. Visual hallucinations occurring alone are almost always suggestive of organic psychosis.

### Attitude to the Hallucinations

The delirious patient is terrified by the hallucinations and tries to escape from them. In acute schizophrenia also the patient becomes anxious and terrified with the onset of hallucinations. In the later stages of the illness when the patient finds out the 'meaning' of the strange happenings and comes to term with his symptoms, there is no more anxiety and anger against his persecutors swaying his emotional field. The chronic schizophrenic is least bothered about his hallucinations. In depression the patient is not terrified by the experience and accepts or even welcomes them as he considers himself worthy of being punished in the described manner.

### 3. Perceptual Disturbances of Time and Space

All sensory processes have a space time dimension and it is never possible to have a sensory experience independent of their spatial and temporal relations. Space and time are universal but how they are experienced (i.e. the 'personal' space and time as against the 'physical' space and time) is subject to alteration with regard to their extent and duration. Also they may vary from one person to another and in many illness conditions.

### Changes in Spatial Perceptions

Objects appear either smaller or farther away in space (micropsia) or bigger and nearer (macropsia or megalopsia). They have been referred to earlier. The space may appear infinite and boundless and objects in the vicinity may recede to infinity.

Retinal diseases produce changes in spatial perception. Oedema produces micropsia. Scarring and distraction produce others. Diseases of accommodation and convergence also alter space perception. Disturbances of perception are however more common in central lesions affecting the posterior parts of temporal lobes and might be the premonitory symptoms of an epileptic fit. They can occur also in delirium and schizophrenia.

### Disorders of experience of time

Awareness of the passage of time is altered in health and disease. In health, pursuit of an activity with interest and absorption gives an awareness that time is fleeting. Monotony of work and idleness produce the opposite effect. Extreme exhaustion may give rise to a feeling that time stands still.

In illness, the anxious and depressed patient reports that the time drags heavily and in states of extreme depression time does not appear to move at all. A day is described as long as an age. Experience of time is deranged in delirium and during epileptic fits, as well as in lesions of the temporal lobe and under the effect of hallucinogenic drugs (e.g. Mescaline, LSD). Time is either 'stretched out' or racing past at a frightening speed. *deja vu* and *jamais vu* are alterations of perception possessing a quality of reminiscence, *deja vu* is the sensation of intense familiarity to objects or situations which the person has never seen earlier, as if the patient had been associated with it throughout in the past. In *jamais vu* even the most familiar situations appear strange and fresh. These may occur at times in normals under severe anxiety but are seen excessively in those with temporal lesions where they might be heralding an epileptic attack.

**Discontinuity of time.** Normally one is aware of the passage or 'flowing' of time. There is no blank or vacuum between two points of experience. Time gaps the interval which is personally observable. However, in some cases this awareness of continuity of time is lost. Two events stand side by side not bridged by the time span. One moment, the person is here and in the next in an entirely new situation with emptiness intervening. This can occur in individual schizophrenic patients.

### Movement

In abnormalities of perception of movement a moving object appears to travel faster or slower. Or movement is perceived in an object which in reality remains stationary.

## Body Image Disturbances

The sense of one's own body with the disposition of its parts in relation to the surrounding world is known as the body image (body schema) against which we can appreciate the postural changes, and soundness and integrity of the body. It is an abstraction acquired during development incorporating physiological (sensory data from exteroceptors, and proprioceptors) and psychological (personality, emotions and social interaction) elements. Thus disorders involving disturbances of body image should be considered in the light of cerebral pathology and psychopathology. A majority of them result from organic lesions, for example, temporal lobe lesions which cause right-left disorientation, sensory inattention, anosognosia (ignorance of the presence of illness specifically of paralysis) or autotopagnosia (inability to recognise any part of the body). In many cases, however, there are associated psychological factors contributing to the genesis of the symptoms and in others such disturbances occur in the absence of brain pathology. The latter would appear not to be true alterations of body schema, but represents faulty experience of the self.

**Phantom limb.** Phantom limb is an example of a distorted body image. It is commonly seen after amputation of a limb, but removal of breast, genitalia or the eye also might trigger phantom phenomena. The member even after amputation remains a subjective reality to the patient with its spatial characteristics and sensations including pain. Lesions of nerve plexuses, brain stem and thalamus at times produce phantom limbs and emotional states of the individual, influence the phantom sensation.

**Autoscopy.** Autoscopy is perception of one's own body image projected into external visual space. It is sometimes called phantom mirror image and occurs mostly in the visual modality alone. It may occur in epilepsy or migraine episodically or in delirium and rarely depression. In negative autoscopy the patient fails to see his image while looking in the mirror. In internal autoscopy the internal organs are visualised while viewing the body.

## Disturbance in the Experience of Self

The experience of 'self consists of (i) awareness of the existence of the body and its activities; (ii) awareness of its boundaries and (iii) knowledge of body's integrity or 'one-ness' at a point of time and constancy over a period of time.

**Depersonalisation.** In depersonalisation the subject feels that he is no more his normal natural self. The physical body seems changed and the identity lost, so that ultimately he appears a stranger to himself. Often this is associated with a sense of alteration in the environment also (derealisation) which then appears to him as alien and unreal. The change is noted in the physical environment but it can involve the interpersonal relationships as well.

**Loss of body boundaries.** The difference between one's body and the rest of the world is learnt in infancy when the child distinguishes between 'me' and 'not-me'. This boundary between the self and the environment (called the ego boundary) is lost in many clinical conditions. The body appeals continuous and merging with the environment at some point which the patient is not able to define. Changes occurring in the factual exterior are perceived to be occurring inside his body and vice versa. Disregarding the physical barrier, thoughts, feelings and actions of other people are directly attributed as his own and controlling him. His own thoughts, feelings and actions become alien to him and are attributed to external agencies who have implanted them through X-rays, radio waves, telepathy and hypnosis in his body. These are passivity feelings or 'made' experiences as the patient thinks that he is the passive agent for such experiences made by outside influences.

## Other Disturbances of Bodily Experience

- *Disturbances of bodily shape.* Body becoming animal like, shrunken and shrivelled up, bizarre and destroyed; body becoming flat so that back and chest touch each other.
- *Feelings of change of position in space.* Body floating in the air or falling down.
- *Reduplication of body parts.* Having two heads, four legs, etc.

- *Change of size.* Affecting the whole body or parts as ears, nose or limbs. Lilliputian experiences (microsomatognosia) where body assumes an extremely small size, or feeling of enlargement (macrosomatognosia). Normal proportions of body may or may not be preserved.

- *Change in mass.* Experience as heaviness, light-weightedness, emptiness (body appearing as a mere framework) and hollowness (food seems to fall into a vacuum).

- *Displacement of parts.* Head and neck not connected; head sinking into body: sexual organs growing from abdomen or from the head.

- *Loss of integrity.* Body fragmented, not staying together.

- *Body parts not alive.* Body appears wooden and skin papery.

### Clinical Significance

As mentioned earlier disturbances of body schema provide for study a fascinating area where organic pathology and psycho-pathology overlap each other. A wide spectra of disorders emerge in an equally wide array of clinical settings. Some of these as heaviness of the body and depersonalization may occur in normal individuals under exhaustion and in sensory deprivation or prior to falling asleep. Minor disturbances are exaggerated by anxiety and hypochondriasis. In delirium, or under the influence of hallucinogenic drugs as 'LSD, Mescaline and Cannabis, distortions of shape, mass and integrity can be seen. Ego boundaries are lost and body appears floating in the air. Episodic neurological illness as epileptic attacks and migraine could produce bizarre symptoms as autoscopy and duplication of body parts and static lesions of the brain might be responsible for symptoms like anosognosia and phantom phenomena. Psychotic illness with no brain damage causes pathological changes in bodily sensations, subjectively indistinguishable from the organically caused types.

### FUNCTIONAL SIGNIFICANCE OF PERCEPTIONS

In spite of his illness the patient is an organising animal and disorganisation resulting in meaninglessness is a condition which he cannot tolerate. The mind integrates and interprets what is received into a meaningful whole—even if the attributed meaning might turn out to be untrue. That is, perceptions are organised and meaningful.

Things seldom are what they appear to be. The need, mental set and, the mood of the perceiver determine what he sees and how. In other words, perceptions are functionally selective. We see things as we are—not as they are.

## FURTHER READING

1. Cutting, J, Principles of Psychopatholgy: Two Worlds—Two Minds—Two Hemispheres. Oxford University Press, 1997.
2. Max Hamilton ed. Disorders of Perception. In: Fish's Clinical Psychopathology. John Wright Bristol, 1976.
3. Sims A. Symptoms in the mind: An introduction to descriptive psychopathology, 2nd ed. Bailliere Tindall, London, 1995.

# 6

# Disorders of Thought

K Kuruvilla, Anju Kuruvilla

Since thinking is perhaps the most important function of the human mind, disorders of thought have always had an important place in the diagnosis of mental disorders. Elicitation of abnormalities in thinking is an important part of the mental status examination, and once thought disturbance is reliably established in a patient, it can assume diagnostic significance.

The term 'thinking' refers to a patient's ideational experience and includes the following three processes:

1. *Thinking concerned with reasoning or mental problem solving.* Normal thinking consists of a goal directed flow of ideas, symbols and associations initiated by a person and leading to reality oriented conclusions. An attentive listener will be able to follow the verbal and ideational sequence of the speech resulting from such thinking.

2. *Thinking dominated by imagination.* This does not go beyond what is rational or possible. It helps in planning out everyday life and solving of anticipated problems as and when they come up.

3. *Thinking dominated by fantasy.* Here there is very little contact with reality. This is also called 'dereistic' or 'autistic' thinking. Fantasy enables one to escape from unpleasant realities, so a person may use it deliberately for a short while. For example, a timid and shy individual may indulge in a fantasy where he pictures himself as a dashing hero who saves a young woman from a group of eve-teasers and thus gets praises from the media and is surrounded by autograph seekers. In some abnormal states of mind fantasy, however,

73

may become a way of life and the individual may find it difficult to differentiate between fantasy and reality.

Spoken words and writings are the main media through which a person's thought process becomes accessible to an interviewer. We often assume that abnormalities in the spoken word are reflective of disturbance in thinking, however, this may not always be so. The ability of congenitally deaf children to think conceptually, though they are not able to speak, is an example of this lack of correlation between thought and language. Similarly there are aphasic patients who may not be able to express themselves through spoken words, but can convey their ideas which are logical and coherent through performance. One also comes across patients who, during a psychiatric interview, exercise conscious control over their language and thereby prevent access to their abnormal thought process. Thus we cannot always conclude with certainty that normal language reflects normal thought process or that a disordered language function is invariably a product of disordered thinking. Yet observation of language function remains the easiest method of evaluating thought process. The term 'thought disorder' is used in this chapter to include both thought and language disorders seen in psychiatric disorders.

Emil Kraepelin emphasized the clinical importance of making careful observations of patient's speech and behaviour in order to arrive at a psychiatric diagnosis almost a century ago. It is important to bear in mind that even the newer diagnostic systems like DSM-5 and ICD-11 are based on this atheoretical but clinically-based observational process. This chapter is an attempt to deal with thought abnormalities in the same way. It focuses on common abnormalities of thought that may be present in persons with psychiatric disorders.

## The Assessment of Disorders of Thought

As mentioned above, in clinical practice, thought disorder is most commonly understood through the patient's conversation with the interviewer, though the patient's writings and non-verbal behaviour may also contribute. The most useful strategy is to encourage the patient to talk freely and unhurriedly on a wide variety of topics. An interview that is too structured, which does not allow the patient to talk, which forces the patient to respond with 'yes' or 'no' answers or one where the interviewer is excessively focused on documentation may fail to elicit thought disorder, even if it is present.

Asking the patient to repeat a simple story in his/her own words after the interviewer has narrated it, making him/her write essays on general topics or encouraging the patient to give his/her opinion on a social or political event may prove to be more effective in bringing out thought disturbances than confining oneself to the standard questions in mental status examination schedules.

If in the early phase of the interview a patient is found to be guarded and evasive in his/her answers to questions aimed at detecting thought abnormalities like delusions, it may be helpful to keep that line of questioning aside for a time and shift to other aspects such as details on the family of origin, educational background, occupational history and marital life. It is not rare to find that the information which the patient was reluctant to part with earlier, is given away while talking about these other topics, at times inadvertently, often because of the improved rapport.

The axiom accepted by all branches of clinical medicine, that examination of a patient is a continuous process from the time he/she walks into the doctor's room till he/she walks out of that place, is of utmost importance in psychiatry especially in the context of the mental status examination (MSE). An alert clinician can pick up evidence of thought disorder even outside a formal assessment. For example, a patient in whom delusions could not be elicited during the formal mental status examination, refused to close his eyes when the clinician asked him to do it as a part of the neurological examination. On enquiry, he explained that his enemies, who were lurking outside the interview room, may rush inside and harm him when his eyes were closed. He also suspected that the doctor himself was making him close his eyes with some sinister motive.

It is advisable to make a verbatim record of the questions put to the patient and his/her responses to them, instead of merely recording the interviewer's inferences. Such a recording will help others who may examine the patient at a later date to assess the validity of the original interviewer's conclusions.

When a clinician recognizes that the speech or writings of a patient are unusual, the context must be taken into account, including the patient's intellectual, educational and cultural background and other symptoms that may be present.

The interviewer also has to be cautious in accepting at face value the responses of the extremely defensive patient who tries to conceal his/her symptoms and the unduly compliant one who admits to every type of thought disturbance that is enquired about. Both these problems can be reduced by avoiding leading questions as much as possible. In situations where a leading question is unavoidable and the patient admits to having a symptom, encourage him/her to describe and elaborate on that symptom in his/her own words instead of accepting 'yes' as an answer. At times one comes across patients with 'iatrogenic' false positive symptoms, many of whom have undergone repeated psychiatric interviews in the past.

While earlier, thought disorder was considered to be pathognomonic of and always present in schizophrenia, it is now understood that it may be present in a diverse variety of clinical conditions in psychiatry, as well as occasionally in people who do not meet the criteria for any psychiatric diagnosis, particularly when they are fatigued or stressed. Given the several different explanations for the various terms used to describe the different thought disorders as well as overlapping concepts, scales such as the Scale for Thought, Language and Communication by Andreasen (1986), have been devised in an attempt to clearly define terms and improve the reliability of assessments.

### Classification of Thought Disorder

It is customary to classify thought disorders into 4 types.
1. Disorders of stream of thought
2. Disorders of form of thought
3. Disorders of possession of thought
4. Disorders of content of thought

### 1. Disorders of Stream of Thought

These are reflected in the quantity, rate of production and quality of speech and include.

**A. Pressure of speech.** A marked increase in the quantity of spontaneous speech is observed. The patient talks very rapidly and it is difficult to interrupt him/her. At times even when interrupted, he/she may continue to talk. Simple questions which could be answered in a few words are answered at great length. Speech tends to be loud and emphatic. This type of speech may be seen in mania or hypomania, stimulant intoxication and occasionally in highly anxious individuals.

**Example**

Interviewer—"Which branch have you chosen for your engineering course?"

Patient—"*What else? I can't think of taking anything other than computer science, a branch which provides tremendous opportunities and has terrific potential for future progress; not only my future, but also everybody's future depends on it, even progress in medical science depends on your knowledge of computer science. My one and only choice was computer science.*"

**B. Flight of ideas.** This is invariably associated with pressure of speech. It is a nearly continuous, high speed flow of speech where the patient jumps from one topic to another. Each topic may be superficially related to the previous one, or an environmental stimulus may bring in quite an unrelated topic. The progression of thought is illogical and the goal is never reached.

**Example**

Interviewer—"When did you start smoking ganja?"

Patient—"*I started it when I was in veterinary college. All students in veterinary college smoke ganja. The veterinary course is more difficult than MBBS. We have to study many more subjects. We learn about every animal, but you know only about man. We have to remember the temperature of sheep, dogs, cats and every other animal. They fail you in practical exams if you don't remember all these.*"

Flight of ideas is a common symptom in mania. When severe, the flight may be so extreme as to make the patient's speech incoherent, as before one thought is completely expressed in words, another thought forces its way forward. Although flight of idea is most commonly seen in mania, it may at times be evident in patients with schizophrenia and organic states.

C. **Loosening of association.**The patient exhibits thought processes characterized by disconnected ideas which seem to jump from one topic to an unconnected topic.

**Example**

Interviewer—"Where did you go?"

Patient—*"I went to the park and bought Raju's tomato home in a bag of books and dolls."*

D.**Circumstantiality.** A pattern of speech that is very indirect and delayed in reaching its goal. In the process of explaining something, the speaker brings in many tedious and unnecessary details, but eventually reaches the goal.

**Example**

Interviewer—"When did you get admitted to this hospital?"

Patient—*"We have been planning to come here for a long time, but my son was getting ready to go back to Dubai. He is working as a cashier in a bank there. He seems to be quite happy there. So we decided to come here after he leaves for Dubai. Meanwhile we met Dr Aravind, whose wife is my uncle's daughter. They had come home on vacation. You know, he did his MD here. Nice chap, very helpful. Even his father is like that. He told me all about this hospital. So we finally decided to come and reached here yesterday morning."*

Circumstantiality may be seen in schizophrenia, obsessional disturbances and organic brain syndromes.

E. **Retardation of thinking.** The train of thought is goal directed, but slowed down. Patient experiences having to make extra-ordinary effort to think about even simple matters. The patient may express this experience in terms of a difficulty to make decisions, poor concentration and lack of clarity of thought. This type of retarded thinking is most typically seen in depressive disorder.

F. **Blocking.** This refers to an abrupt interruption in the train of speech before a thought or idea has been completed. After a period of silence lasting from seconds to minutes, the speaker indicates that he/she cannot recall what he/she has been saying. Presence of thought block should be inferred only if patient is able to describe the loss of thought as the reason for pausing and not based on the clinician's observation alone.

## 2. Disorders of Form of Thought

A. **Poverty of thought.** This often manifests as poverty of speech. Spontaneous speech is very restricted. Though the patient responds to questions, the answers tend to be brief, concrete and unelaborated. If not prompted, additional information is rarely given. Replies may be monosyllabic and some questions may be left unanswered.

**Example**

Interviewer—" What is your complaint?"

No response.

Interviewer—" What brought you to this hospital?"

Patient—*"Headache."*

Interviewer—"What else ?"

No response.

Interviewer—"Do you have any trouble other than headache?"

Patient—*"Sleep."*

Interviewer—"What sort of difficulty you have in sleeping?"

Patient— *"Not good."*

B. **Poverty of content of thought.** The patient gives long replies to questions and there is no dearth in the quantity, however it carries a little information. Language may be vague, abstract, repetitive and stereotyped. As a result of this, the interviewer finds that though the patient has been answering the question for quite some time, he/she has not given adequate information.

**Example**

Interviewer—"What do you plan to do after the completion of your studies?"

Patient—*"Yes, of course I must complete my studies. I should do it as soon as possible, within the shortest time possible. My future depends on that, in fact everybody's future depends on what he or she does. No doubt it is important in my case also. It is time that I do something about it. No doubt, I must take steps in that direction."*

The term 'alogia' is used for the impoverishment of thinking seen both in poverty of thought and poverty of content of thought.

C. **Tangentiality.** The patient tends to wander away from the intended point, moving further and further away, never returning to the original idea. If asked, the patient may not even remember the original point. Authors like Andreasen (1979) restrict the term tangentiality to deviations to answers to questions and do not apply it to deviations in spontaneous speech, thus differentiating it from derailment.

**Example**

Interviewer—"Why are you chosen by God to receive these special messages?"

Patient—"*As a believer in God, I have to do my duty. Whatever happens, the communication system must go on. If you stop one method of communication another will start because God is everywhere and listening to us. That means this conversation is heard throughout the universe.*"

D. **Derailment.** This is an abnormality in spontaneous speech in which ideas are found to slip off to another one that is only obliquely related or even completely unrelated. The pattern of speech sounds often disjointed. Some writers include loosening of association, tangentiality and even flight of ideas under the term derailment.

**Example**

The interviewer narrates the 'Donkey and Salt' story and asks the patient to tell that story in his own words.

Patient—"*A merchant used to go to the market with his donkey. The donkey used to carry cotton clothes. But the number of times she had to go up and down depends on the weight of the stolen property. On the return trip there was no weight because it was salt. Too much of salt is not good for the body and it has to be eliminated.*"

E. **Incoherence.** It is a pattern of speech that is incomprehensible. A set of words and phrases appear to be used together arbitrarily without any logical connection or respect for rules of grammar. It is also known as 'word salad' and may resemble 'jargon aphasia' seen in organic brain disease. It may occur along with derailment, but is to be distinguished from it; in derailment the loss of connection is between large units of speech such as sentences, whereas in incoherence the abnormality is within the sentence itself with words and phrases joined meaninglessly.

**Example**

Interviewer—"What was the reason for the quarrel between you and your brother?"

Patient—*"It started with a two feet by four feet iron piece without any conclusion or enquiring they have been contacting the Inspector of Police without any authority before they could give a boxful of medicines and the flask for use till noon."*

F. **Illogicality**. This refers to thinking which contains erroneous conclusions or internal contradictions. It may take the form of the patient arriving at an inference that is unwarranted or illogical.

**Example**

*"Cement is necessary to build temples and operation theatres. So operation theatre is a temple. In operation theatre there is light, light for the doctor. In temple also there is light. So God is the doctor there."*

G. **Clang associations**. The patient's choice of words is determined by their sound and not by their meaning. This often leads to use of redundant words and reduces intelligibility of speech. It may lead to punning and rhyming and is often seen in manic patients.

**Example**

Interviewer—" How do you feel today?"

Patient—*"I feel happy, happy like a puppy. Puppies and hippies irritate my papa. He may pop off one of these days."*

H. **Neologism**. The patient uses new words of his/her own whose derivation cannot be understood. The patient uses these words to covey some specific meanings or ideas, but these are not understandable to others.

**Example**

Patient—*"All my colleagues are involved in 'vigitilo' against me. As I was coming to the hospital, my fellow passengers were doing 'vigitilo' in the bus."* Further discussion with the patient enabled the interviewer to understand that for the patient the term 'vigitilo' meant an international conspiracy to harm him.

I. **Word approximation**. Commonly used words are used by the patient in a new or unconventional way. Often the meaning may be evident, though the usage may be peculiar or bizarre. Sometimes word approximations may manifest as the use of stock words.

**Example**

Patient—*"The psychiatrist who treated me at Madurai gave me 'tablet metro'. When he found that it did no good, he gave me 'electric metro'. Before that I used to have 'natural metro' with leaves and roots from an Ayurvedic doctor."*

J.  **Echolalia**. A pattern of speech in which the patient echoes or repeats the words or phrases of the interviewer.

**Example**

Interviewer—"What work did you do today?"
Patient—*"What work did you do today?"*
Interviewer—"Did you help your mother in the kitchen?"
Patient—*"Did you help your mother in the kitchen?*

K.  **Stilted speech**. Speech is said to be stilted when it is excessively formal in character. The patient may sound excessively polite, pompous or archaic.

**Example**

Patient—*"A visit to this renowned seat of medical knowledge and dedicated service has been contemplated by me and my beloved family for a considerably long period. Despite our single minded efforts to bring that desire to fruition earlier, it became a reality only now due to monetary and other adverse expected and unexpected difficulties."*

L.  **Self reference.** The patient tends to bring in some relationship to himself, whatever the subject under discussion may be.

**Example**

Interviewer—"What time is it?"
Patient—(Looks at his watch and says) *"Seven o'clock. That is my problem. I never know what the time is. May be I should keep better track of the time."*

M. **Paraphasia.** Here the patient uses wrong words in his statements, despite adequate vocabulary and education. There are two types of paraphasias: (a) Phonemic and (b) Semantic.

In **phonemic paraphasia,** sounds or syllables slip out of sequence and result in wrong expression. In common parlance this is called spoonerism.

**Example.** *"I want to boil my icicle"* (instead of "I want to oil my bicycle").

In **semantic paraphasia,** patient is found to include an inappropriate word in his / her attempt to express a specific idea. Commonly this is referred to as 'malapropism.'

**Example.** *"The personal atrocities* (instead of 'attributes') *of my boss have immensely contributed to the growth our company."*

N. **Stereotypy.** This is a needless, constant repetition of speech or action in many different settings, irrespective of the context. When stereotypy is manifested as a constant repetition of a word or phrase, it is called **'verbigeration'.**

**Example**

Patient—*"I took mathematics for B.Sc. My ambition was to become an engineer. I took mathematics. My family's financial situation was not good. I took mathematics. The job I am doing has nothing to do with mathematics. I took mathematics."*

O. **Perseveration.** Perseveration is the persistence of a response to an earlier stimulus even after a new stimulus has been presented. It is often associated with organic brain disease.

**Example**

Interviewer—" What medicines have you been taking to control your fits?

Patient—" *Gardenal and Eptoin."*

Interviewer—"Are they helping you?"

Patient—*"Gardenal and Eptoin"*

Interviewer—" Are you experiencing any side effects from these medicines?"

Patient—*"Gardenal and Eptoin"*

### Abnormalities of form of thought in schizophrenia

At one time disturbances in the form of thought were considered to be pathognomonic of schizophrenia. Recent studies have shown, however, that many of these abnormalities may be seen in other functional psychoses, as well as in organic states. Formal thought disturbance is considered to be the result of an underlying disturbance in conceptualisation, particularly in schizophrenia. Two types of disturbance in conceptualization are seen in schizophrenia. viz. (a)concreteness and (b) over-inclusiveness.These abnormalities can be elicited in the clinical setting by simple tests which the clinician himself/ herself can administer.

a. **Concreteness.** The formation of a concept involves abstracting a common feature from a group of objects. Goldstein and Scheerer (1941) showed that patients with brain damage or schizophrenia are often unable to abstract and operate mostly at the concrete level.

Clinically, the presence of concrete thinking can be demonstrated by asking the patient to group a collection of objects according to their common features. For example, if six objects such as pencil, button, scissors, comb, key and hammer are given, the normal individual is likely to group the scissors, key and hammer together since they are made of metal, the button and comb together as they are made of plastic and keep the pencil by itself away from the other two groups. Many brain damaged patients and some patients with schizophrenia are unable to do this.

Another clinically useful test is asking the patient to interpret common proverbs. A proverb is a concrete representation of a general principle. While normal persons can explain this general principle, patients with impairment of abstract thinking cannot go beyond the words used in the proverb in spite of their intelligence and education.

**Example**

A patient having a Master's degree in English literature gave the following interpretation for the proverb 'all that glitters is not gold'—

*"It means, all that appears to be gold need not be gold. Gold is not the only substance which glitters, there are materials like silver, stainless steel, glass, etc. which also glitter."*

People who are unfamiliar with proverbs or unable to interpret them may be asked to describe the differences and similarities between items such as an apple and an orange or a table and a chair. A response regarding similarity as 'round' to the first question would suggest concreteness, while a response of 'fruits' would suggest adequate abstraction. Similarly in the second example, a response of 'furniture' indicate a satisfactory abstraction instead of 'both have four legs'.

It is important to bear in mind that impairment of abstract thinking is not specific for schizophrenia and that there are those with schizophrenia whose ability for abstract thinking is intact.

In addition to concreteness, proverb interpretation by a person with schizophrenia may also demonstrate bizarreness, personal references and a tendency to use a larger number of words to express an idea that necessary.

**Example**

A patient's response to the proverb 'barking dogs seldom bite'
Response:"*A dog which bites does not move, a dog that is not able to smell can never move. A dog is able to feel and touch, it makes use of all the five senses. What is the spelling of dog? D- O -G. Can you reverse it? It becomes G-O-D, God. So dog and God are the same. There ends the circle. Every one treats me like a dog, but I know God is within me.*"

b. **Overinclusiveness.** Payne (1962) and Costello (1970) have pointed out that some patients, especially those with schizophrenia, are unable to preserve the boundaries of their concepts and so their concepts become abnormally vague and ill defined. Features which are normally only remotely related to a concept become integrated to it.

The patient's interpretation of proverbs may show evidence of such overinclusiveness.

**Example**

The proverb 'birds of the same feather flock together' was interpreted as follows by a patient—

"*People with the same characteristics join together and they also make a lot of noise like birds when they are together.*"

Over-inclusiveness can also be tested by asking the patient to group a number of blocks of various sizes, shapes and colours, based on varying concepts.

**Example**

A patient with schizophrenia made the following group-ings—

3 groups according to shapes.

4 groups according to colour.

In the second trial, he put all the blocks together in a single group. The patient explained the basis of this as , *"I can touch them all."*

Third time he made 2 groups—one group consisting of all circles and triangles and explained as, *"These go together because they represent women. Circles stand for their pottu (bindi) and the triangles stand for female genitalia."*

All the other blocks were put together without any explanation.

### 3. Disorders of Possession of Thought

Normally a person experiences his/her thinking as his/her own, although this sense of personal possession is never in the foreground of his/her awareness. He/she also has the feeling that he/she is in control of his/her thinking. In some psychiatric conditions, there is a loss of control or sense of possession of one's own thinking.

Loss of control of thinking may manifest as thought passivity, where the patient experiences his/her thoughts being under the control of other forces.

The loss of possession of thought may take one or more of the following forms:

a. **Thought insertion**. The patient knows that an external agency is inserting thoughts in his/her mind and he/she recognizes them as not his/her own.

b. **Thought withdrawal**. The patient feels that as he/she is thinking, the thoughts suddenly disappear and they are withdrawn from his/her mind by an external force.

c. **Thought diffusion**. The patient knows that as he/she is thinking, everyone else is thinking in unison with him/her or he/she is certain that everyone else is participating in his/her thoughts. He/she may also experience that thoughts escape his/her mind and are heard by everyone else. This experience may be labelled **'thought broadcasting'**.

Fish (1967) used the term 'thought alienation' as a general term covering all the three experiences described above. Taylor and Heiser (1971) opine that experiences of influence and experiences of alienation should be considered as different entities. In experiences of influence, the patient knows that the thoughts are his/her own, but believes they are controlled or imposed upon by some external agency. In contrast, in experiences of alienation, the patient believes that the thoughts are not his/her own, but are coming from an outside source.

While in the past, the above disturbances of possession of thought were considered to be pathognomonic of schizophrenia, recent studies have shown that they may occur in other conditions as well.

## 4. Disorders of Content of Thinking

a. **Mystical Experiences.** This can occur in normal people under certain conditions, for example, during induction phase of general anaesthesia or during intense religious experiences. It may also occur transiently in patients with schizophrenia. The distinctive characteristics of mystical experiences are: (i) The subject finds it difficult to express or describe it to someone who has not experienced it (ii) the person feels that the mystery of the universe has been suddenly revealed to him (iii) the mystical experience itself may last only for a very short while, but the individual finds it unforgettable and treasures the memory (iv) a feeling that the experience has occurred under the influence of a superior power and the subject himself/herself is only a passive recipient of it (v) a sense unity with the superior power.

b. **Fantasy.** A fantasy is a mental experience that is recognised by the subject as unreal, but is still expected or hoped for. Fantasy may be (a) **creative fantasy** which prepares a person to some later action or (b) **daydreaming fantasy** which is a response to wishes that cannot be fulfilled. Although daydreaming tends to diminish with psychological and biological maturation, to some extent it persists throughout life. In autistic and borderline psychotic individuals, day-dreaming occupies a major part of the person's wakeful hours and impairs the capacity for normal relationships and responsibilities. Pseudologia fantastica or pathological lying is a condition where the person believes in the reality of his/her fantasies intermittently, during which time, he/she acts on it also.

c. **Phobia.** An exaggerated and pathological dread of a specific object or situation resulting in a compelling desire to avoid the feared object or situation. The sufferer is aware of the irrationality of his/her reaction. Phobic reactions may occur in a wide variety of situations like crowded or enclosed spaces, vehicles, heights, animals, seeing blood, etc.

d. **Obsessions.** An obsession may be defined as a thought, image or impulse which keeps on recurring in a person's mind, overriding internal resistance. In other words, when an obsession occurs in a person's mind, he/she is unable to get rid of it even though he/she realises it is senseless and wants to get rid of it. The person recognizes that these thoughts, impulses or images are a product of his or her own mind and does not believe these are imposed from without, in contrast to 'thought insertion.' Obsessional images can be very vivid and at times can be mistaken for hallucinations. Obsessive ruminations may centre around any sort of topic. An obsessive rumination may be followed by a compulsive act. An obsessive impulse may manifest itself as a wish to touch, count or even carry out antisocial or self-injurious acts. Obsessions occur in obsessive compulsive disorder and may also be seen in depression, schizophrenia and some organic brain diseases.

e. **Ideas of Reference.** When a person ascribes personal significance to neutral remarks or comments, he/she is said to be having 'ideas of reference'. This may occur in normal individuals in social situations which make them self-conscious. In psychoses the experience is very frequent.

f. **Overvalued idea.** A basically acceptable and understandable, sustained false belief, maintained less firmly than a delusion, yet it preoccupies the person to the extent of dominating his/her life. Apprehension based on an over-valued idea is given undue probability and attempts to deal with it pursued beyond reason.

**Example.** *The dysmorphophobic patient assumes he/she attracts attention because of a real or assumed bodily defect and avoids all social contacts.*

g. **Delusion.** Delusions are considered central to psychoses and reflect an abnormality of thought. A simple definition states that a delusion is a false belief based on incorrect inference of external reality, firmly held despite evidence to the contrary and not shared by the person's culture. However, there have been many different definitions that have been proposed over the years. Consistencies that have been identified among various definitions include the description of delusion as an abnormal belief, that is considered false based on logic and rational thought or abnormal as not shared by the culture he/she belongs to, which is fixed and unalterable despite evidence to the contrary and is held in clear consciousness in the presence of an intellect that is adequate to evaluate the evidence. Additionally, the individual may give grossly abnormal explanations for his/her belief, and may act on these.

There are several methods of classifying delusions. One customary way is to classify them as primary and secondary delusions.

**Primary delusions.** In a primary delusional experience, a new meaning is attributed to an apparently unrelated psychological event. Primary delusions are often considered to be pathognomonic of schizophrenia, though may be found occasionally in other conditions as well.

**The appearance of a primary delusional experience may occur in 3 stages.**

1. Delusional mood: The patient is aware that something is going on around him/her that concerns him/her, but does not know exactly what it is.
2. Delusional perception: A new meaning is attributed to a normally perceived object. How the patient arrived at this new meaning cannot be understood in the light of his affective state or previous attitudes.
3. Delusional idea. The delusional perception leads to a sudden delusional understanding of the meaning of all what has been going on.

**Example.** *A young medical student had been feeling that something fishy and strange was going on in the college and hostel over the last few months. One day he observed one of his classmates picking his teeth with a pencil. Suddenly, the patient 'realised' that everyone around him considered him a homosexual.*

Primary delusional experiences are commonly seen in acute schizophrenia, but when the disorder become chronic, they often get buried under the mass of secondary delusional misinterpretations.

**Secondary delusions.** These are delusional experiences arising from and understandable in the light of the morbid experiences of the patient. These may be seen not only in schizophrenia, but also in other psychotic conditions.

**Example.**

*A man with erectile dysfunction sees his wife talking to another male in the neighbourhood and comes to the conclusion that she is having an extra-marital relationship. When the husband returns home after work if the wife is found to be unkempt, it is because "she no longer cares for my (husband's) feelings". If she is well dressed, it is "to impress the other man".*

Types of delusions based on the content.

Content of delusions are influenced by the patient's social, cultural and educational background. Based on the content, delusions are classified into the following groups.

**a. Delusions of persecution.** The patient believes that he/she is being harassed and cheated, that others are trying to kill her, trying to poison her food, or indulging in witchcraft/conspiracy to harm her and her family. Persecutory delusions may take the form of **'delusions of reference'**. For example, on seeing people talking to each other or laughing, the patient comes to 'know' that they are talking ill of her or laughing at her. These may occur in schizophrenia and mood disorders. A patient with delusions of persecution may believe that it is only he who is being poisoned or subjected to witchcraft. The influence of education and socio-cultural factors may be evident in the contents of delusions, with the patient from a rural background believing that he/she has become a victim of black magic while the urban patient reports delusions of being subjected to hypnosis, telepathy, radio waves or spy satellites. It is interesting to note that with the increasing exposure to movies, television programmes and easy access to mobile phones, for the rural population, the difference in the content of delusions between rural and urban patient is fast disappearing in India also, as it happened in the West in the last century.

b. **Delusions of jealousy.** This usually presents as delusions of marital infidelity, and also between partners in live-in relationships, both heterosexual and homosexual. The patient may misinterpret every activity of his/her partner, as a confirmation of his/her delusion and even torture the partner to extract a 'confession'. This condition is also called 'Othello' syndrome after the central character in Shakespeare's famous play with the same name. This may occur in schizophrenia, delusional disorder, affective psychoses, alcohol dependent syndrome and organic delusional sates.

c. **Delusions of love.** More often seen in women than in men, here the patient is convinced that a person who usually is of a socially superior position, is in love with her, although the alleged lover himself would never have talked to her or even be aware of her existence. The patient may pester the 'lover' with frequent phone calls, repeatedly sending letters and gifts, etc. This delusion is also known as 'erotomania' or 'de Clerambault's syndrome'.

d. **Delusions of grandeur.** The patient has markedly exaggerated notions about his/her own importance: Exalted birth, possessing immense wealth, extraordinary abilities and knowledge or supernatural powers, being chosen by God for some special mission. Though common in mania, it may also be seen in schizophrenia, and organic conditions like general paralysis of insane.

e. **Delusions of ill health.** The patient has a delusion that he/she is suffering from a serious illness like cancer, AIDS, etc. It may also take the form where the patient believes that a foul odour is emanating from him/her, some part of his/her body is abnormal in shape or size, his/her brain or some other part of the body is infested with parasites. Such delusions may be seen in depressive disorder, schizophrenia and delusional disorder (when it may be referred to as a monosymptomatic hypochondriacal delusion).

f. **Nihilistic delusions.** The patient denies the existence of some of his/her organs, his/her mind and sometimes his/her whole body itself. He may deny his existence as a person and say he is dead. This is most commonly seen in depression, but may also occur in schizophrenia.

g. **Delusions of guilt.** A self reproachful and self critical attitude is common in depression, but in severe depression this may take the form of delusions of guilt, when he/she believes he/she is the worst sinner, that he/she has not only ruined his/her family, but is also responsible for all calamities that are happening in the world.

h. **Delusions of poverty.** This type of a delusion is seen more commonly in depression, when the patient falsely believes that he/she is impoverished. He/she may even refuse treatment because he/she does not want to worsen the family's poverty by making them spend money on him/her.

i. **Delusional misidentification.** It is seen in 2 forms.

   1. **Capgras phenomenon:** The patient believes on the basis of a delusional perception, that a person who is very close to him/her is replaced by an imposter. He/she accepts that there is a great similarity between the familiar person and the imposter in appearance; yet he/she is certain that they are different people. This symptom may be seen in persons with schizophrenia, mood disorder and organic brain disorders.

   2. **Fregoli phenomenon:** A familiar person whom the patient believes is his/her persecutor, assumes the guise of a stranger. This symptom may be seen in schizophrenia.

Types of delusions, historically considered to have high diagnostic value.

1. **Bizarre delusions.** This term is used when a delusion is totally implausible and absurd, not understandable and does not derive from ordinary life experiences.

While in DSM IV, this one symptom of having bizarre delusions was given special importance in the diagnosis of schizophrenia, in DSM 5 this special significance was removed due to poor reliability in distinguishing bizarre from non-bizarre delusions.

**Example.** *"The patient believes that 4 invisible microwave towers have been built in his village and aliens from Mars are controlling all his movements through these.*

2. **Systematized delusion.** A delusion is said to be well systematized when the central theme of the delusion is extensively developed and conclusions are so logically deduced from the premises assumed, that a coherent and connected organization of ideas is established.

**Example.** *A person is convinced that his wife's parents are trying to kill him. The warm welcome he received when he visited their house is interpreted as an attempt to cover up their evil intent. His mother-in-law compelled him to have lunch there in order to poison him. The abdominal pain he developed that evening was the result of the poison. Two days later, when the father-in-law spoke to the patient's wife over the phone, he enquired about the patient; that was to check whether the poison has worked.*

Systematized delusions are frequently seen in delusional disorders, while they are uncommon in schizophrenia.

Types of delusions based on congruence with mood.

a. **Mood congruent delusion.** A delusion which is in keeping with the prevailing mood of the patient.

**Example.** *A severely depressed woman believed that her past sins were responsible for the devastation caused by the tsunami in their village and kept falling at the feet of passersby to apologise to them.*

b. **Mood incongruent delusion.** A delusion not in keeping with the patients mood which cannot be understood as arising from that mood state.

**Example.** *An elated, manic patient believing that a microchip is planted in his brain and his thoughts are controlled by his enemies.* Current diagnostic and classificatory systems are highly dependent on the clinical features that are elicited through history taking and mental status examination. Among the various manifestations of psychiatric illnesses, disturbance of thought process is of paramount importance in facilitating our understanding of the nature and type of the disorder a patient has. So time and effort spent in the elicitation of thought abnormalities will prove to be worthwhile both in clinical practice and academic pursuits.

## FURTHER READING

1. American Psychiatric Association. Diagnostic and Statistical Manual of Mental Disorders. 5th edition, Washington, 2013.

2. Andreasen NC. (1979). Thought, Language and Communication Disorder. Archives of General Psychiatry, 36, 1315–1330.

3. Andreasen NC. (1986). Scale for Assessment of Thought, Language and Communication. Schizophrenia Bulletin, 12:3: 473–482.

4. Butler RW and Braff DL (1991). Delusions: A Review and Integration. Schizophrenia Bulletin, 17:4: 633–647.

5. Casey P and Kelly B. (Eds). Fish's Clinical Psychopathology, signs and symptoms in psychiatry. 3rd edition, London:Gaskell, 2007.

6. Costello CG. Classification and Psychopathology. Pp 1–26 in CG Costello (Ed) Symptoms of Psychopathology. New York. Wiley, 1970.

7. Goldstein L and Scheerer M. (1941). Abstract and concrete behaviour—an experimental study with special tests. Psychological Monographs,53:2, 1–151.

8. Kochler K. (1979). First rank symptoms of schizophrenia. Questions concerning clinical boundaries. British Journal of Psychiatry, 34,:236–248.

9. Payne RW. (1962). An object classification test as a measure of overinclusive thinking in schizophrenic patients. British Journal of Clinical and Social Psychology.1:213.

10. Rao AV and Kuruvilla K. Psychiatry. BI Churchill Livingstone, New Delhi, 1997.

11. Sadock BJ and Sadock VA. (Eds.) Synopsis of Psychiatry, 10th edition. Lippincott, Williams and Wilkins, Philadelphia, 2007.

12. Sadock BJ, Sadock VA and Ruiz P (Eds.). Comprehensive Textbook of Psychiatry. 9th edition. Lippincott Williams and Wilkins, Philadelphia, 2009.

13. Sims A. Symptoms in the Mind, 3rd edition. Saunders, London, 2003.
14. Taylor MA, Heiser JF. (1971). Phenomenology. An alternative approach to diagnosis of mental disease. Comprehensive Psychiatry.12:480.

This picture was drawn by a 29-year-old man diagnosed as suffering from schizophrenia when a piece of paper and sketch pen were offered to him. When asked what the picture was about the reply was as bizarre and incomprehensible as the picture itself indicating fragmentation of thought and incoherence. The picture further shows stereotypy and symbols with personal meaning.

# 7

# Clinical Evaluation of Disorders of Mood and Affect

C J John

Affect is the feeling tone pleasant or unpleasant that accompanies an idea. This is the prevailing emotion tone during the interview, as observed by the clinician. The term mood is used for an emotion state which usually lasts for some time and which colours the total experience of the subject. Thus while an affect is a short-lived response, a mood state is a lasting disposition. The variation of mood states in every day life situation, when appropriate is normal. To understand abnormal affective states, a preliminary distinction in the following way is useful.

a. Those affective states which emerge in an understandable fashion from some experience even though they appear exaggerated and heavily coloured. Yet depending the severity, the distress caused to the individual and others, the mood state will qualify for an appropriate clinical diagnosis.

b. Those affective states which defeat understanding and arise endogenously as psychologically irreducible. Explanation can only point to biological causes. This distinction helps us to distinguish normal home sickness, for instance from excessive but understandable home sickness characterized by aggressive behaviour of a child in a boarding school, and both these from a depression without such causative factor in the environment.

The expression of affect also depends on the cultural factors and the vocabulary available to emotion expression. The predominance of somatic symptoms like aches and pains colouring the depression of an Indian patient from a rural background is documented and is attributed to the sociocultural expectation about what doctors consider an illness and their own evaluation of symptoms as meriting the label of sickness. Thus emotional distress becomes readily expressed in somatic language so that medical treatment is available. Careful evaluation of affect, when interpreted along with the global presentation of the psychiatric symptoms, can be of great help in formulating the final diagnosis of a case.

## CLINICAL EXAMINATION OF MOOD

Disturbance of mood manifests not only at an ideational level but will be evident in the general behaviour and appearance of the patient. In depression, the feeling of misery is often evident by facial expression and bodily movements. The characteristic physiognomy of the depressive has facial lines running down and outwards from the furrow to the drooping mouth. The body may be generally flexed and the hands often wrung, in some patients there is a purposeless agitation, while in others there occurs a slowing, sometimes to the point of immobility. Weeping, sighing, and brief expostulations of distress such as "God help me" "I am suffering" are not uncommon in depression. In manic patients the passion for movements is evident from his aimless movements for sheer sake of moving out of delight. Often a manic is overdressed with colourful garments and will show the enhanced well-being by way of cheerful expression or will be at the peak of feelings of excessive power or by irritability and anger towards others. There will be excessive liking for social relationships and he will open spontaneous conversation with even strangers. In anxious patients there will be a pressure of movements with an aim to seek peace, trying to get rid of something. He may be fidgety and sits at the edge of the chair with trembling fingers making the inner distress very evident. A shake hand with him will reveal the cold and clammy skin of the person suggesting autonomic arousal.

Thus the examination of mood starts right from the moment the patient appears before you for evaluation. The objective data one gathers, need to be supplemented with additional enquiries about the subjective mood state of an individual.

Replies to such probing will reveal hidden thoughts of guilt, worthlessness, somatic concerns, suicidal intent or plans arising from an underlying mood disorder. The patient should be encouraged to describe his feelings in detail, in his own words. It is mandatory to enquire about suicidal idea in everyone who has a depressive mood and assess the risk. The doctor should also assess whether the patient is masking his true feelings. The subjective mood state may not be always in keeping with the observed behaviour due to denial of the inner distress, or due to incongruous emotional expression.

Systematic evaluation of mood state can be carried out in the following fashion.

## 1. Range of Affect

To accurately express the patient's full affective capacity or range of emotionality, the doctor must cover a diversity of topics in a flexible way. The dominant emotion demonstrated is likely to be related to patient's prevailing mood state. However, the doctor must be certain that the interview includes varied subject matter, to find out whether the patient shows a constriction or limitation of affect. In major depressive disorder, the affect of individual is usually restricted to depression only. But in dysphoric states and dysthymic disorder the interviewer can appreciate that there is a normal range of affective responses depending upon the content of the topics. Before commenting on the constriction of affect, the doctor should also make a note of the cultural differences existing as far as outward expression of affect is concerned.

## 2. Intensity of Affect

In normal expression of affect, there is a variation in facial expression, tone of voice, the use of hands, and body movements. The consideration in assessing intensity of affect is in evaluating how much of emotion is expressed, as judged, by the above parameters. Terms like blunt, shallow, flat and intense refer to the depth of the affect expressed. Patients with histrionic personality disorder often shown intense emotional responses. The other extreme is lack of depth of affective responses seen in some chronic schizophrenics. To diagnose flat affect, one should find virtually no signs of affective expressions and the face is usually immobile. The patient is fully conscious and oriented, sees, hears observes and remembers, but he lets everything pass by him with the same total indifferences and remains dead with wakeful eyes.

### 3. Changeability of Affect

This is also related to the range of affective responses the patient has and the mobility of facial muscles. The consideration here is whether or not the affectivity is in an appropriate way according to the variation in topics discussed in the interview. It is important to introduce various topics to assess the changeability of affect. In some drug induced states, e.g. antipsychotics like chlorpromazine, trifluoperazine, halo-peridol, resperidone, the expression of mood may be masked due to extrapyramidal side effects. In Parkinsonism also, this can occur, resulting in mask-like facies.

### 4. Appropriateness of Affect

The appropriateness of the patients emotional response can be considered both in the context of the topic the patient is discussing and in the context of the interview situation. A schizophrenic patient may exhibit silly giggling, weeping spells or spells of laughter, which may be evoked without any understandable reason. A patient may start laughing as he narrates the story of death of a close relative which is an incongruous affective response to the idea expressed. Some discuss inappropriateness in relation to the situations and incongruity to ideation level. In either case, its presence points to an abnormal psychological disturbances.

### CLASSIFICATION OF EMOTIONAL DISORDERS

Frank Fish classifies emotional disorders in the following manner.

1. Abnormal emotional predispositions.
2. Abnormal emotional reactions.
3. Abnormal expressions of emotion.
4. Morbid disorders of emotion.
5. Morbid disorders of the expressions of emotion.

## 1. Abnormal Emotional Predispositions

*Disposition* refers to the affective state with which a person habitually confronts himself. Such dispositions are partly determined by childhood experiences. There are certain people who are emotionally cold, indifferent, lack emotions, and shows absence of finer feelings. It has been suggested that maternal deprivation in early childhood may be a factor in such personality traits. Due to maternal deprivation or a lack of bonding with a caring person in early childhood, the individual is deprived of caring and loving experience and hence develops such a predisposition. Those who are subjected to various types of abuses in childhood, especially child sexual abuse are predisposed to intense emotional outbursts and lack of emotional control as they grow as adults. Another type of abnormal predisposition is proneness to mood swings like happiness or sadness. Depressive personality disorder is characterized by a pervasive pattern of depressive cognition and behaviors. Cyclothymic disorder is a chronic and non-psychotic state characterised by alternative periods of euphoric mood and depression. Some of them have vulnerability to develop certain types of psychiatric disorders. For example, persons who are cyclothymic are vulnerable to develop bipolar disorder in later life.

## 2. Abnormal Emotion Reactions

A normal person is able to withstand the effects of external stimuli and preserve an emotional balance. But each person has his breaking point. The type of emotional reaction depends upon the individual's personality and the intensity of traumatic situation. The common reaction to a loss is depression and threat is anxiety. But when this exceeds the normal limits one speaks of abnormal reactions. One can go into exaggerated states of normal fear, the acute anxiety states. Anxiety is a disagreeable emotional state in which there are feelings of impending danger, characterized by uneasiness, tension or apprehension. There is an accompanied anticipation of something untoward happening. It is also characterized by autonomic nervous system discharges like altered respiration, increased heart rate, pallor, dryness of mouth and dilated pupil. Musculoskeletal disturbances like trembling and weakness also can occur. Some differentiate anxiety from fear, as in the latter there is a real conscious external danger present. Anxiety according to psychoanalysis stems from unconscious inner conflict. Panic is an acute intense anxiety feeling accompanied by diorganisation of personality and function. A panic attack is characterized by a discrete period of intense fear or discomfort developing abruptly and reaching a peak within minutes. There are associated somatic signs that indicate a hyperactive autonomic nervous system.

Whenever psychological adaptive mechanisms threaten to decompensate, anxiety appears. It may appear in chronic low grade form as a constant accompaniment of life. Sudden changes in life situation may evoke an increase of anxiety or precipitate an episode of panic as a warning that more disastrous emotional decompensation may result. The presence of generalized anxiety or occurrence of anxiety attacks is not always an indication of one clinical entity, but is rather a psychosocial signal of danger that can occur in any diagnostic category of physical or emotional disease. Free floating anxiety is the nucleus and key symptom of generalized anxiety disorder. Anxiety and depression become major symptoms in stress related and adjustment disorders. Anxiety triggers the avoidance reactions in the phobic disorder.

### 3. Abnormal Expression of Emotion

These are emotional expressions, the behaviour very different from expected normal reaction. To state this in simple terms, the anxiety reaction to threat or depressive reaction to loss is conspicuously absent. The anxiety may be denied purposely by some, in an attempt to put on a bold face, even when anxiety is actually felt. Thus, the normal emotion is dissociated. Such phenomenon can occur in conversion disorder and is termed the *la belle indifference*. The hysterical person will complain of loss of functions, e.g. paralysis of limbs, but will maintain a normal emotional response. Fish defines perplexity as an abnormal expression of emotion. It is state of puzzled bewilderment, with mild clouding of consciousness and can occur in anxiety and in pre-psychotic disorder when new strange psychotic symptoms are emerging.

## 4. Morbid Disorders of Emotions

This includes emotional disorders which arise without an understandable cause. Morbid sadness is the vital component of major depressive disorders, and this abolishes the normal reactive changes of emotion or emotional resonance. Morbid depression is associated with diurnal variation, loss of energy, loss of libido, lack of appetite, weight loss, and early morning awakening. Morbid depression can be differentiated from stress induced depressive disorders and dysthymic disorders, by the presence of reactivity, early insomnia, and the tendency to get better in the presence of pleasing company. There will be a lot of associated features accompanying morbid depression. There will be loss of drive, and all experiences are considered from the worst negative aspect. Normal activity is carried out with a sense of difficulty and incompetence against a background of inner unrest, loss of self confidence and lack of pleasure in living. Morbid anxiety can occur as a symptom of depression, especially in those depressions where agitation is a vital component. There is, however, no one-to-one relationship between inner feelings of anxiety and degree of agitation. Thus some extremely anxious depressives are almost mute and stuporous because their intense anxiety paralyses all voluntary actions.

Morbid mood changes like euphoria occur in the manic phase of bipolar disorder. Euphoria refers to the first moderate level in the scale of pleasurable affects. It has been defined as a positive feeling of emotional and physical well-being. Elation is characterized by an air of enjoyment and increased self-confidence with associated motor overactivity. Exaltation is extreme elation, and is usually associated with delusions of grandeur. It merges into ecstasy which represents a peak state of rapture. In mania all this range of affective responses can occur and are completely unmotivated. In contrast to depression, there is a lack of response to depressing influences and everything is seen in the best possible light. This primary derangement in mood state may lead to faulty judgement and disinhibited behaviour. There are other associated features like increased pressure of speech, overactivity to the point of exhaustion and tendency to be argumentative. The person may claim extra power, and unrealistic abilities. Often the affective response merges into one of *irritability*, when the person may exhibit a chronic diffuse state of anger. In the absence of specific disturbance in affect or mood, the patient is described as *euthymic*.

There can be affective changes in certain organic states, the most important one meriting mention being the Temporal Lobe Epilepsies. A wide variety of ictal mood changes, which are short lived and are characterized by depression, anxiety, euphoria and ill-defined unpleasant feelings are reported. Elation can occur in General Paresis of Insane, but lacks its infectious quality and rarely is associated with flight of ideas. Silly euphoria, lack of foresight and general indifference are found in frontal lobe lesions, particularly when the orbital surface of frontal lobe is affected. In multiple sclerosis there is often an element of euphoria.

Morbid disorders of affect can occur in schizophrenia also, when the emotional disturbance like anxiety or depression stems from the thought disturbances and other hallucinatory experiences of schizophrenia. Prodromal affective changes can occur before the evolution of core schizophrenic symptomatology. There can be impoverished and inappropriate emotional responses like silly gaiety in schizophrenic illness.

Certain drugs can cause disorders of emotions, and this has to be kept in mind while evaluating a person. Antihypertensive like alpha methyl dopa, propranolol and clonidine can cause depression. There are many more to this list. Steroids given exogenously can cause a physical well-being and sometimes elation or even psychosis.

### 5. Morbid Disorders of Emotional Expression

The emotional expression in schizophrenic may be grossly abnormal, and is often qualified as 'blunted' or 'apathetic' affect. The marked insensitivity to finer aspects of social relationships and the inappropriate silly euphoria are abnormal emotional expressions arising out of a morbid psychotic state. Such abnormalities are seen in certain depressives also as in the 'smiling depressives'. They, when overwhelmed by miseries can produce a communicating smile and they stand a high risk for suicide. Such depressives are often noticed to be smiling with their lips, but not with their eyes, so that despite their apparent cheerfulness there is lack of movement of the muscles around there eyes. A little probing into depressive ideation in such patients will evoke overt depression with weeping spells.

Affective lability is a state wherein the patient has difficulty in controlling his emotions. Morbidly depressed individuals may have such problems, and even the slightest stress may move them to tears. Lability of affect can occur in certain abnormal personalities and also in manic states and organic states. In affective incontinence, there is complete loss of control and there is a sudden expression of emotions in the absence of any adequate cause. This symptom while present is indicative of an organic pathology and can occur in cerebral arteriosclerosis and multiple sclerosis. Episodes of 'forced laughing' or 'forced weeping' attributed to a lack of control occur in coarse brain diseases.

**CONCLUSION**

Clinical evaluation of mood is an important aspect of psychiatric examination. One of the vital considerations in synthesizing the clinical symptomatology will be in ascertaining whether the disorder is primarily due to the derangement of mood, or secondary to other morbid processes. This has an important clinical significance, and helps in differentiating the affective disorders from other psychiatric disease like schizophrenia. Even when affective disturbances are elicited as part of schizophrenia, it has prognostic significance. Apathy denotes poor prognosis and mood states like depression or anxiety, if prominent in the schizophrenic process suggest a good prognosis. Clinical depression is common in the medically ill and is associated with impaired quality of life, decreased compliance with medical treatment, and increased morbidity and mortality. Careful evaluation and documentation of affective disturbance thus becomes crucial not only in every psychiatric disorders, but also in all medical illnesses.

# 8 The Assessment of Insight and Judgement in Psychiatry

K P Abdul Salam

Assessment of insight and judgement is extremely important in clinical interviews as it helps reaching a diagnosis. There are not many scales available to rate these two aspects in patients. The very nature of the topic at hand makes it essentially a clinical endeavour. Therefore, it is imperative that clinicians learn to assess judgement and insight through clinical methods.

## INSIGHT

Insight, in a clinical sense, is often defined as the extent to which the person is aware of one's own illness. Clinically, this is especially important when psychotic symptoms are present. Absence of insight is one of the first clinical cues that one is dealing with a 'non-neurotic' disorder. Absence of insight is a hallmark of schizophrenia and other psychotic disorders and bipolar affective disorder mania. In the so-called "neurotic" disorders, the person usually has insight into the illness. In such cases, it is usually the person himself/herself who seeks treatment, whereas in other disorders, most often, the person is brought for treatment by family or significant others.

*Ms. B., 27-year-old married female, Engineer, working for an international company, higher socio-economic status; pre-morbidly had paranoid personality traits, presenting with 2 years duration of doubting her husband's fidelity. Her difficulties recently flared up when she recently saw a red mark on her husband's body which she believed were due to amorous activities. The first clue regarding absence of insight into the illness came when she requested treatment for her husband so that he could be 'straightened out'. She wanted the treatment team to 'counsel' her husband so that he wouldn't engage in immoral activities again.*

A very direct question, "Do you think you have an illness/ a problem?" might give an idea about the presence of insight. However, during clinical interview, it's important to listen to the way the person explains his/her experiences. When someone says, "I *feel* I'm being controlled", most often (though not always), insight is preserved. When insight is absent, the experiences are *real* for the person and are not just *feelings*. Therefore, these are usually framed by the patient in terms such as "I'm being controlled by my mother", "My leg move without me wanting to do it".

*Mr A, 32-year-old male, accountant, working in a private firm, middle socioeconomic status, pre-morbidly, well adjusted; currently presenting with complaints of ten days duration of sleeplessness, irritability and a complaint that, "others are mixing poison in my food". When interviewed, he complained that his neighbours were mixing some poison in his food. He was sure that they were doing it but was unsure of their motives to do so. He couldn't sleep for the last ten days once he "found this out". This is an example of insight being absent.*

Another important clue regarding the person's degree of insight is the readiness to accept and follow the treatment prescribed. A person with complete insight into his/her illness is expected to co-operate in the process of treatment and adhere to the treatment prescribed by the professional. Non-cooperation in the treatment process is an important clue to poor insight on the part of the patient. However, caution should be exercised since some of the resistance towards treatment could be due to factors other than insight such as socio-cultural beliefs regarding modes of treatment and misunderstandings and misinformation regarding side-effects of treatment, for example.

It should also be noted that insight is not affected in psychiatric disorders alone, some medical-neurological disorders could also present with lack of insight. A careful clinical interview and physical examination is therefore warranted.

## Rating of Insight

A clinically useful method of rating insight is in terms of "complete, partial and absent insight". Complete insight is when the person accepts the fact that he's ill. Insight is considered "absent" when the person denies that he's ill. The person, therefore, believes that his mother is *actually* controlling him from her grave and doesn't even accept that it's a 'feeling'; it's a reality for him/her. "Partial" insight is when the person has some degree of awareness into the illness and reluctantly accepts the fact that he's ill. Some patients might have their insight fluctuating so that they accept that they have illness in the morning and deny it in the evening.

*Ms. C, 36-year-old married female, housewife, middle socio-economic background, pre-morbidly, well adjusted, she presented with episodes of being 'unresponsive', 'irrelevant talk' and headache. She was diagnosed to have mixed dissociative disorder. Her brother had passed away a year back but during the episodes of 'irrelevant talk', she used to say her brother was coming back from the Gulf states to meet her and she wanted to go to the airport to receive him. During the initial interview, when she was allowed to calm down and talked to in detail, she gradually came to accept the fact that her brother is no more. However, during a second interview, on the very next day, she again claimed that her brother was still in the Gulf country and that all who believed that he's dead 'were mad'. This case provides an example for fluctuation of insight into the presence of an illness.*

Two related terms are that of "emotional" and "intellectual" insights. Intellectual insight is said to be present when the person is aware of being ill on an intellectual level but this insight doesn't lead to any alteration of behaviour. Emotional insight, on the other hand, leads to the person being aware of the motives behind his behaviour and applies this knowledge to bring about changes in his/her own behaviour.

An elaborate grading of insight involves grading it on six levels:

| | |
|---|---|
| Grade I | Complete denial of illness |
| Grade II | Slight awareness of being ill |
| Grade III | Awareness of being ill but attributes it to factors external to him |
| Grade IV | Awareness of being ill and attributes it to his own dynamics, thinking and behaviours |

Grade V  Intellectual insight

Grade VI  Emotional insight

It can be seen that these gradations and ratings of insight is influenced by some of the early schools of thought such as psychoanalysis. However, a clinical assessment of insight at least on the lines of 'complete-partial-absent' is an essential component in arriving at a psychiatric diagnosis.

*Mr. E., 56-year-old male, sales tax practitioner, middle socio-economic background, premorbidly well-adjusted; presented with complaints of one year duration that other sales tax practitioners in the town were 'preventing him getting new cases'. He believed that they were influencing his clients through mind control techniques and therefore, he was losing business. The look on the face of the practitioner in the next building 'confirmed that this was the case'. During the interview, when the impossibility of such things was gently pointed out, he accepted that he had a mental illness and he was sure that 'other practitioners in the town had done something to make him mad'. This is an example of Grade III insight where he accepts that he has an illness but attributes it to external things.*

*Mr. D., 43-year-old married male, advocate by profession, from middle socio-economic status, pre-morbidly had anankastic traits, presenting three months history of excessive washing and checking rituals. He was diagnosed to have obsessive compulsive disorder— Mixed. His obsessions were related to fear of contamination/germs and he used to engage in washing compulsions in response. He had a fear of his house being looted and hence the checking rituals. He was perfectly aware that these were 'unwanted thoughts' but couldn't help it. He continued to engage in his compulsions though he would accept that 'it was a little too much'. This is an example of intellectual insight, without true emotional insight.*

As for the symptomatology, insight varies in different disorders. The assessment of insight, thus, could be an important tool in the process of differential diagnosis. As discussed above, the presence or absence of insight helps in distinguishing between the "psychotic" and "neurotic" disorders in general. Hallucinations and delusions are usually associated with an absence of insight. The very diagnoses of these two phenomena require absence of insight as an important criterion. When the person has insight into hallucinations, it is considered 'pseudo-hallucination' and not treated as a psychotic symptom in the strictest sense.

On the other hand, there are symptoms which are usually considered 'neurotic', but occur in the absence of insight. Dissociative disorder is one such example. In dissociative disorders, it is presumed that the person 'doesn't know what he/she is doing'. If the person does know what he/she is doing, i.e. if the insight is preserved, factitious disorder would be more favored. Obsessive compulsive disorder is another disorder where insight plays an important role. OCD is a disorder where insight could be present or absent. Absence of insight is considered to be a poor prognostic factor in OCD. Personality Disorder is a similar category where insight could be present or absent. Cluster 'C' personality disorders (avoidant, anankastic and dependant) usually have insight preserved. In Cluster A and B personality disorders, it might be absent, transient or fluctuating. In other diagnoses, the patient might have an intellectual insight while emotional insight at the time of presentation is rare. Habit and impulse control disorders, paraphilias, gender identity disorders are examples of this.

## JUDGEMENT

Judgement is the ability to assess a given situation adequately and act/behave appropriately. Judgement is assessed both through clinical observation and tests. A good clinical interview can give an idea of the person's social and personal judgement.

### Test, Social and Personal Judgement

Test judgement is assessed through some simple verbal tests. Some common questions used to this end are:

1. What will you do if you see a sealed, stamped and addressed envelope lying on the ground?
2. What will you do when your house is on fire?
3. What will you do when you see a man lying on the ground?
4. What will you do when you are late for your job?

Answers like, "I will open the envelope and read the letter inside", "I will sit and enjoy the colours of the fire", and "I will kill the man", "I will resign from the job" etc. are indications of poor judgement.

Signs of poor social judgement could be obtained from the case history. Instances such as attacking someone suspecting that he/she was a private detective, getting naked in the public, getting overtly sexual on the road, etc. are signs of poor social judgement. Poor social judgement can be inferred from clinical observations too. Disinhibition and overfamiliarity seen in mania, for example, is a result of poor social judgement. A patient coming to the clinic and asking for the files to be shown 'since he's an inspector from the Department of Health' is another example.

*Ms F., 28-year-old unmarried female, unemployed, from lower socioeconomic status, pre-morbidly well adjusted was brought with the complaints of excessive and irrelevant talk and restlessness. She was diagnosed to have bipolar affective disorder—current episode manic with psychotic symptoms. The symptoms started a month back when she started claiming that the priest in her village was in love with her. She started believing that there were young males who were walking around her house 'just to get a glimpse' of her. When she was brought in for the interview, she did not sit in the designated seat but wanted to sit in the chair of the clinician as that would 'fit her demeanor'. She also wanted to 'wrap her arms around the clinician's shoulder' and 'be friends'. Impairment in social judgement is obvious from clinical observation itself in such patients.*

Personal judgement is usually assessed through questions concerning the person's future plans. If the person's future plans are in accordance with the person's social, economic and educational background, judgement is considered preserved. A person with no formal education saying, "My future plan is to be the Head of Department of Psychiatry" suggests poor personal judgement.

*Mr G, 57-year-old married male, employed as a security officer, lower socio-economic status, pre-morbidly, well-adjusted; presented with 3 months duration of believing that he had supernatural powers. He believed that he could control the 'American media' and that the President couldn't make any move without his permission. When asked about his future plans, he 'was thinking of talking to the Chief Minister to discuss some personal matters'. Personal judgement is clearly impaired in this patient. He was diagnosed to have other non-organic psychotic disorder.*

Thus, judgement and insight are two important aspects to be assessed in clinical interviews. It helps in ruling in and out diagnoses. Therefore, it is crucial that clinicians learn the art of assessing these clinically.

# Neurological Assessment of Psychiatry Patients

Bangalore N Gangadhar, Naren P Rao

## INTRODUCTION

Rapid advances in neurosciences have blurred the boundary between neurological and psychiatric disorders. With better understanding of the neurobiology of psychiatric disorders, the mind-brain dichotomy stands challenged. Also, underlying brain abnormalities for psychological and behavioural manifestations of psychiatric disorders are being increasingly recognized. Conceptually, the distinction between organic and functional basis of psychiatric disorders are becoming thin and likely, artificial. However, clinically it is still useful to recognize the behavioural manifestations of known neurological syndromes for optimal diagnosis and management. Another objective of neurological assessment for a psychiatrist is the examination of *soft neurological signs*—minor neurological abnormalities indicating non-specific cerebral dysfunction without a focal lesion. In this chapter we deal with both these aspects of the neurological assessments.

### History

A detailed clinical history is critical for evaluation of neuropsychiatric patient. Certain indicators in the history can give vital clues to the presence of an underlying focal neurological lesion or an identifiable neurological syndrome, like: an abrupt onset of symptoms, absence of identifiable psychosocial stressors, headache with projectile vomiting, periods of loss of consciousness, altered or fluctuating consciousness, history of seizures, disorientation, urinary/faecal

**115**

incontinence, fever and head injury. A detailed history with specific emphasis on age and status of siblings and parents, and presence of family history of any degenerative disorders or epilepsy needs to be collected.

**Higher mental functions:** It is useful to follow a standard order for assessment of higher mental functions as it could give a clue to the interpretation of deficits and avoid misdiagnosis. For example, in a patient with impaired attention, examination for impairment in memory is invalid. Specific emphasis needs to be given for the examination of consciousness, attention and concentration, speech and language. Other features of higher mental functions like memory, perceptual disturbances, insight and judgement are not described here as they are essential components of standard mental status examination and described elsewhere in the book.

*Consciousness:* Consciousness involves arousal and content. Arousal denotes the level of awareness and is primarily dependent on the projections from ascending reticular activating system, brainstem and thalamus to the cortex. Lesions of this pathway results in alterations in arousal and coma-like state which may mimic psychogenic unresponsiveness. *Akinetic mutism* is characterized by mutism, inability to move limbs but preserved consciousness. In some patients, extraocular muscles and pupillary reflexes are spared. Some patients will have emotional outbursts as well. Lesions of projections from ascending reticular activating system result in akinetic mutism. Another similar disorder, *locked in syndrome*, results from an upper pontine tegmental lesion. The patient with locked in syndrome cannot speak, swallow and is paralysed. However, the vertical eye movements are preserved and they can indicate using eye movements.

*Attention and concentration:* As attention is central and basic requirement to other cognitive functions, it is first among other cognitive functions to be tested. Digit span test (DST), in which the subject is asked to repeat a random string of numbers presented at the rate of one per second, is a simple but useful assessment of attention. A forward digit span of less than five in DST is considered impaired attention. Concentration, the ability to sustain attention, can be tested bedside by asking the patient to recite the months of the year or days of the week backwards. Random letter cancellation test is a simple but effective way of testing concentration. In this task the subject is presented a series of random letters and asked to tap the desk or cancel the letter whenever the target letter (for example, A) is read out. Omission, commission and perseveration errors indicate an underlying organic cause. In unilateral attention/ hemi-neglect, the patient is able to recognise the stimulus when presented to the contralateral side. However, when the stimulus is presented simultaneously to both ipsilateral and contralateral sides the patient is unable to recognise.

*Language:* Similar to attention, language is required for effective communication and hence for examination of other cognitive functions. Language functions include speaking, listening, writing, reading as well as miming (sign language). Perisylvian regions are involved in language functions; Broca's area is important for speech production and Wernicke's area is important for reception. These two areas are connected by the Arcuate fasciculus. An acquired deficit in language function which can impair production or comprehension of language is called *aphasia*. Aphasia is classified into fluent aphasia and non-fluent aphasia. Commonly used aphasia tests include assessment of comprehension, naming and repetition. Comprehension is tested by asking patient to carry out simple requests like closing or opening eyes. Repetition is tested by asking the patient to repeat short phrases and naming is tested by asking patient to say names of common objects. Non-fluent aphasia is characterised by minimal telegraphic speech, impaired repetition with relatively preserved comprehension. Lesions of the Broca's area, area 44 in the dominant hemisphere, results in such deficits. Fluent aphasias are caused by damage to Wernicke's area or the arcuate fasciculus. It is characterised by high rate of word production, paraphasias, neologisms, impaired comprehension, and omissions of grammar. They are subdivided into anomia, transcortical/isolation aphasia and conduction aphasia. In anomia the patient has inability to name the objects and in conduction aphasia, the patient has lost the ability to repeat a sentence but has preserved comprehension and speech production. In transcortical aphasia, the patient has lost the ability to produce or comprehend language but has preserved repetition and often able to repeat even lengthy, complex sentences.

## Cranial Nerves and Eyes

One has to follow the same method of examination as in neurological disorders. Certain findings which are of relevance to psychiatry need to be specifically looked for. Lack of vision is a common finding and one needs to differentiate psychogenic vision loss from loss due to organic etiology. Thorough assessment of visual fields by confrontation method is required to identify known patterns of visual loss like bitemporal hemianopia or quadrantonopia which will help locate the site of lesion. A patient with dissociative disorder may complain of tubular vision loss whose dimensions will remain the same even after increasing the distance of the target object from the eye (*tunnel sign*). On the other hand, the patient with organic tubular vision will have increase in dimension of visual field with increase in distance (*funnel vision*). Eye movements need to be examined in detail—both rapid and slow eye movements are to be checked along with size and shape of pupil. Light and accommodation reflex can give clues regarding the underlying aetiology; Argyll Robertson pupil, described as absence of light reflex with intact accommodation reflex along with irregular pupil and atrophy of iris, is characteristic of neurosyphilis. Wernicke's encephalopathy is characterised by ophthalmoplegia and nystagmus; chronic alcohol dependence is a strong risk factor.

## Examination of Motor System

The motor system examination includes examination of tone, bulk and power of muscles and eliciting superficial reflexes and deep tendon reflexes.

*Weakness*: Weakness due to neurological conditions follows a characteristic distribution and pattern; (a) upper motor neuron (UMN) (b) lower motor neuron (LMN) (c) neuro-muscular junction (d) muscle disease. In UMN type of weakness there will be increased tone, increased deep tendon reflexes and pyramidal pattern of weakness characterised by weak extensors in upper limbs and weak flexors in the lower limbs. UMN weakness also prominently affects distal and finer movements. Babinski reflex (plantar) is classically extensor in the UMN type of weakness. LMN type of weakness is associated with wasting, fasciculation, decreased tone and absent reflexes. Neuromuscular junction weakness is characterized by fatigable weakness, normal or decreased tone and normal reflexes. Muscle diseases are associated with wasting, decreased tone and preserved stretch reflexes. The weakness is more in the proximal muscles than distal muscles.

*Tone*: Abnormalities in muscle tone could give an indication to the site of lesion. While LMN and cerebellar lesions result in reduced tone (flaccidity), UMN lesion results in increased tone (spasticity). Extrapyramidal syndromes like Parkinson's disease are characterized by cogwheel rigidity. Bilateral frontal lobe damage results in *gegenhalten*, which is also seen in catatonia.

*Abnormal involuntary movements*: Examination for abnormal movements are of particular importance to psychiatrists. Dystonia is a sustained muscle contraction with twisting movements or maintenance of abnormal postures. Focal dystonia can occur independently as in writer's cramp, blepharospasm or could be antipsychotic-induced. Tremor is a regular, rhythmic oscillating movement around a joint. Parkinson's disease is characterised by rest tremors, cerebellar lesions by intentional tremors and metabolic encephalopathy is associated with postural tremor. Myoclonus is a jerky movement and is associated with Creutzfeldt-Jakob disease and Hashimoto's encephalopathy. Asterixis is sudden lapse in muscle contraction when the patient is actively attempting to maintain posture. It is not typically seen in psychiatric conditions, and when present indicates an organic disorder. Nocturnal myoclonus could be an early sign of clozapine associated seizure and warrants early investigation. Tics are associated with Obsessive compulsive spectrum disorders and when present have important treatment implications for the comorbid psychiatric condition.

*Reflexes:* Both tendon reflexes and superficial reflexes need to be checked. Being an objective part of the examination, the reflexes can give clues to identify the nature of weakness. Examine the tendon reflexes (biceps, triceps, supinator, knee, ankle) as well as the superficial reflexes (abdominal and plantar). Exaggerated reflex is suggestive of UMN lesions, whereas absent reflex is suggestive of LMN lesions. A pendular knee reflex is classically described in cerebellar lesions.

*Gait:* Gait is a co-ordinated action requiring integration of sensory and motor functions. Ask the patient to walk and observe posture, arm swing, whether the gait is symmetrical or not and the pace of walking. Patients with dissociative disorder often present with gait ataxia. One of the commonly described gait impairments is atasia-abasia; the patient staggers, appears as if he is in great danger of falling but catches the railings, furniture or the examiner at the last moment. Patients may show signs of fear and distress on standing up, tend to sway at the hips and when they fall, they fall en-mass. Some patients may drag their leg, whereas in true hemiplegia, the patient will swing their paretic leg outward with a circular motion (circumduction).

## Sensory System

Sensory examination should be done with specific emphasis on peripheral neuropathy and posterior column involvement. Examine for individual modalities—vibration, joint position, touch, pain and temperature. While the sensory examination is less reliable even in healthy individuals, the pattern of deficits can give a clue to psychogenic basis for the deficit. For example: (a) loss of sensations with abrupt splitting in the midline indicates psychogenic basis as sensory fibres of the skin normally spread across the midline (b) inconsistent patterns of sensory loss like loss of sensation over entire face without involvement of scalp (c) discrepancy in type of sensory modalities lost, like loss of pain sensation but preserved temperature sensation (d) absence of sensory loss when the affected limb is kept out of patient's sight.

## Primitive Reflexes

These responses give important clues regarding the dysfunction of frontal lobes. These are seen in elderly individuals without any frontal lesion, but when present in young individuals suggest frontal lesions. Below is a list of common primitive reflexes. Unilateral primitive sign may point to ipsilateral frontal pathology.

| Reflex | Procedure to test | Positive sign |
|---|---|---|
| Snout reflex | Gently tap the lips | Pouting/pursing of the lips |
| Rooting response | Gently stroke the angle of the mouth | Pouting and tendency to follow the stimulus |
| Glabellar tap | Tap the glabella repeatedly | Continued blinkin |
| Grasp reflex | Stroke the palm | Tendency to grasp the fingers |
| Groping reflex | Show an object to the patient | Tendency to grasp and follow the object |
| Palmomental reflex | Stroke the thenar eminence of each hand separately | Contraction of mentalis muscle on the same side |
| Corneomandibular reflex | Touch the cornea with a cotton whisp | Movement of lower jaw |
| Tonic foot response | Stroke the heel | Tonic grasp of the toes similar to grasp reflex |

## Neurological Soft Signs (NSS)

These are minor neurological abnormalities indicating non-specific cerebral dysfunction. A number of motor and sensory tests are employed to examine NSS. A near normal intelligence and absence of focal neurological disorders are considered a prerequisite to assess NSS. They are traditionally reported to lack specificity, validity or localizing value. A number of scales have been developed to assess NSS—Neurological Evaluation Scale, Quantified Neurological Scale, Physical and Neurological Examination for soft signs and Cambridge Neurological Inventory. These scales are a collection of individual tests which measure sequencing of complex motor movements, extraocular movements, motor coordination, sensory integration and primitive reflexes. These signs are seen in different psychiatric conditions and well documented in schizophrenia. Some examples of neurological soft signs are given as follows.

| Neurological soft sign | Description | Positive sign |
|---|---|---|
| Tandem walk | Ask the subject to walk in a straight line, heel to toe | More than 2 missteps/ grabbing/falling before completing distance 12 feet |
| Stereo-gnosis | Ask the subject to identify the object placed in his/ her hand with eyes closed by feeling the object. Two trials with two objects | Unable to identify both objects |
| Grapha-esthesia | Ask the subject to identify the number written on the tip of his/her finger with eyes closed. Write two numbers | Unable to identify both numbers |
| Fist-ring test | Ask the subject to place his/her hand on the table in the position of a fist and in the position of a ring alternately. Ask the subject to repeat 15 times. | Major disruption of movement or complete breakdown of motion or more than four fist/ ring confusions |
| Fist-edge-palm test | Subject is asked to touch the table with edge of hand, side of fist or palm in rhythmic sequential pattern | Major disruption of movement or complete breakdown of motion or more than four confusions |
| Ozeretski test | Ask the subject to place both hands on the table. One hand is placed with palm down and other hand in the shape of a fist. Ask the subject to simultaneously alternate the positions | Major disruption of movement or complete breakdown of motion or more than four confusions |

Contd.

Contd.

| Neurological soft sign | Description | Positive sign |
|---|---|---|
| Rhythm tapping test | Subject is asked to *reproduce* a series of taps with eyes closed | More than one error |
| Finger thumb opposition | Ask the subject to touch individual fingers with thumb | Major disruption in movement or more than 4 confusions |
| Synkinesis | Ask the subject to follow an object with his head still—move the object in horizontal gaze | Movement of the head even when they are told to keep it still |
| Finger nose test | Ask the subject to touch his/her tip of the nose with tip of his/her index finger with eyes closed | Marked tremor or past pointing |

## Related Higher Cognitive Function Tests

The mental status examination reflects the integration of cortical functions. However, individual lobes have specific functions and can be tested by individual tasks. While traditionally considered functions of higher cortical regions, studies have shown that subcortical lesions also can result in some of these deficits.

*Apraxia*: It is an acquired disorder of learned, skilled and sequential motor movements. It is a disorder of motor planning with intact low level motor functions like strength, co-ordination, sensation and comprehension. Different kinds of apraxia are described. *Ideomotor apraxia* is characterised by the inability to perform previously learned motor acts. It is tested by asking the patient to follow simple verbal commands: (a) to blow out a match or protrude a tongue (buccofacial apraxia) (b) to flip a coin or salute (limb apraxia) (c) to bow or to stand like a boxer (apraxia of whole body movement). *Ideational apraxia* is inability to perform complex motor tasks that involves a sequence of related but separate steps. The subject may be able to perform individual steps of the sequence of tasks but are unable to do the complete sequence. It is tested by asking the subject to perform sequence of tasks like 'open the toothpaste and hold it in one hand, then take the toothbrush and hold it in another hand, and now place the toothpaste on the toothbrush'.

*Right–left disorientation*: It is the inability to distinguish right from left on oneself and in the environment. Ask the subject to show a body part on the right or left side or ask the patient to point to right or left body part of the examiner, to examine right–left disorientation. While of limited value when seen in isolation, it is of importance if seen along with other features of Gerstmann's syndrome.

*Finger agnosia*: It is the inability to recognize, name and point to individual fingers on oneself and on others. It is tested by asking the patient 'what is the name of this finger' while showing the index finger of examiner. Nonverbally it can be tested by a two-step procedure. In the first step, ask the subject to close his/her eyes and touch one of their fingers. In the second step, ask the subject to point to same finger on examiner's hand. Lesions of the dominant parietal-occipital lobe are most likely to cause finger agnosia.

*Constructional ability*: It is the ability to draw or construct two dimensional or three dimensional figures. It is tested by asking the patient to (a) reproduce two and three dimensional drawings like a diamond, cross or box (b) asking patient to draw a picture like clock, on command. Inability to perform on tests of construction are strongly suggestive of parietal lobe lesions.

*Alternating sequences—visual pattern completion test*: This test examines the ability of the patient to alternate between two visual patterns. Provide the patient with a stimulus figure having alternate visual pattern (for example, circle and cross) and ask the patient to reproduce the stimulus figure and then, to continue the alternating sequence. A loss of sequence or perseveration suggests lesion of the frontal lobe. The motor equivalent of this test, fist-palm-side test and fist-ring test have been described under neurological soft signs.

## Neurological Examination of a Patient with Dissociative-Conversion Disorder

The aim of neurological examination in a case of dissociative-conversion disorder is to assess whether the deficit is suggestive of a known neurological syndrome or not. Even if psychiatric disturbances or psychosocial stressors are evident in the patient, one needs to do a thorough examination and a cautious interpretation. When a deficit doesn't adhere to patterns of neuroanatomy or if symptoms are grossly fluctuating/inconsistent, one needs to consider the possibility of dissociative disorder.

A patient with dissociative-conversion disorder can present with varied symptoms which may mimic neurological illness. The following signs and symptoms will help one to differentiate the dissociative-conversion disorder from organic illness.

- Non-anatomic distribution of deficits: The deficits may violate the normal laws of neuroanatomy. For example: (a) weakness in arms and legs along with loss of vision in the ipsilateral eye and hearing impairment in the contralateral ear (b) weakness in ipsilateral upper and lower limbs, without involvement of cranial nerves as seen in true hemiplegia (c) weakness of proximal and distal muscles which do not follow known patterns of UMN lesion.

- Absence of voluntary effort: When asked to demonstrate the weakness or to make a voluntary effort to move the limbs, the person, instead of contracting the required muscle groups, may contract antagonistic muscle.

- Face-hand test: When the "paralytic" hand is raised and left to fall on the face, it may fall slowly or the patient may momentarily display sufficient strength to avoid it from falling on the face.

- Hover's sign: When patient is asked to lift the unaffected leg, the paretic leg is pressed down and when asked to lift the paretic leg, the person will not press down the unaffected leg.

- Abductor sign: The patient will reflexively abduct the paretic leg when asked to abduct the unaffected leg.

- Give-way effort: When asked to carry out an activity, the patient offers brief exertion before moving back to the apparent paretic position.
- Gait disturbances: Patient may show signs of fear and distress on standing up, sways the hips on doing Romberg's test, reels from side to side, falls en-mass without attempting to gain back the posture, astasia-abasia (described above).
- Sensory disturbances: Midline splitting of sensory disturbance (described above), absence of pain but preserved temperature sensation, patchy sensory loss not corresponding to distribution of a peripheral nerve or nerve root like loss of sensation in face but preserved in the scalp, absence of Romberg's sign even with loss of joint position sense, tunnel vision.

### Neurological Syndromes Mistaken for Psychiatric Conditions

A few neurological syndromes can have bizarre clinical presentations and be misdiagnosed as psychiatric disorders. It is essential for a psychiatrist to be aware of these syndromes to avoid the misdiagnosis.

*Charles Bonnet Syndrome:* In this syndrome, complex visual hallucinations occur in the background of macular degeneration. The syndrome is typically seen in elderly individuals. Patients report visual hallucinations of vivid images of scenery, animals or people. Patients have preserved insight into the phenomenon and are not distressed by these images. Also, many patients can voluntarily stop their hallucinations.

*Alien hand syndrome:* This syndrome is characterised by an affected limb performing autonomous complex movements against the patient's will. In certain intermanual conflicting activities, the affected limb may act against the purposeful movement of the other. Grouping of objects are also characteristically seen. Lesions of corpus callosum and medial frontal lobe results in this syndrome.

*Balint's syndrome:* Inability to see more than one object called as simultanagnosia is the characteristic feature of this syndrome. Simultanagnosia is often accompanied by ocular apraxia (inability to direct voluntary eye movements) and optic ataxia (inability to reach objects guided by vision). Biparietal damage, occipital and thalamic lesions are reported to cause simultanagnosia.

## CONCLUSION

Physical examination, and in particular neurological evaluation, is an indispensable part of psychiatric work up. This helps in the early detection of a frank neurological syndrome that could present with psychiatric symptoms. A detailed neurological examination can guide the choice of investigations. Detecting a coexisting neurological condition will help in choosing treatments optimally; for example, avoiding electroconvulsive therapy if there is evidence of intracranial space occupying lesion. No psychiatric examination is complete without a thorough neurological examination.

## FURTHER READING

1. Buchanan RW, Heinrichs DW. The Neurological Evaluation Scale (NES): a structured instrument for the assessment of neurological signs in schizophrenia. Psychiatry Res. 1989 Mar; 27 (3) : 335–50.
2. Butler C, Zeman AZ. Neurological syndromes which can be mistaken for psychiatric conditions. Journal of Neurology Neurosurgery and Psychiatry. 2005 Mar;76 Suppl 1:i31–38.
3. Kaufman MD. Clinical neurology for psychiatrists. 6th Ed. Saunders, Philadelphia, 2007.
4. Sanders R, Keshavan MS. The neurological examination in adult psychiatry: From soft signs to hard science. The journal of neuropsychiatry and clinical neurosciences 1998; 10; 395–404.
5. Strub RL and Black WF. The mental status examination in neurology. FA Davis company, Philadelphia 2000.

# Psychiatric Evaluation of Children

George Isaac *

## INTRODUCTION

Psychiatric evaluation of children is the cornerstone on which all treatment efforts for an emotionally distressed or behaviourally troubled child is built. The capacity for children's psychiatric evaluation stands at a very incomplete stage presently, yearning for research breakthrough to shed light on the problems of children. As it stands today, it is a process that heavily relies on what can be observed and understood by interpersonal interaction, and as such, almost entirely on the capacity of the clinician to observe, elicit information, and come to an understanding. The limitations of our perceptive capacities limit this process, to the observation and interpretation of epiphenomena only in most children today. The ardent hope is that the advancement of technology, especially in molecular biology, genetics, functional brain imaging, computer science, and related areas will soon add dimensions that will make the evaluation a more scientific and definitive endeavour serving as a prelude to more effective, even curative treatment measures. Until such a glorious scenario materializes, we will have to mostly rely on our observational capacities, interpersonal skills, and under-standing of normality and pathology in mental functioning and behaviour to conduct the best evaluation possible.

The psychiatric evaluation of children in the Indian setting cannot indiscriminately follow the formats used historically in many western countries, especially the methods that were heavily psychoanalytic. Until a few decades ago the writings

**129**

on evaluations of children, the bulk of which had been from the United States, had a strong psychoanalytic bias, a format which is not significantly applicable in the Indian context, and by this time has become irrelevant in the west also. During the past two decades there has been an appreciable shift, to direct the evaluation geared towards arriving at an internationally acceptable diagnostic understanding and a less speculative formulation. Hence, such evaluation formats have great relevance to the Indian setting also, though there is obviously a need to modify the process to the Indian context.

Anyone who is experienced in evaluating and treating children in both the East and West, cannot but be impressed by the common thread of humanity children everywhere have inherited and partake in. There is more common to the biology and longings of children everywhere, compared to their differences. This chapter takes into account those common ingredients—biological, psychological, and social of the human child in an international sense, but is primarily intended for the Indian child and clinician in the diverse Indian context, with the child in Kerala being the central focus.

In this chapter the term child is used to represent the preschool and elementary schoolchild as well as the adolescent, except where a specific mention is made of the child at a particular age group or developmental level to point out something unique about the child at that particular group or level.

The evaluation of children differs from that of adults in many obvious and not so obvious ways. Almost always, a child is brought for evaluation by the parent or parents or someone who is the guardian, because of their concern about the child's behaviour, distress, or functioning. Occasionally an adolescent may initiate a consultation on his or her own because of personal concerns. In all cases the information given by the parents play a crucial role, setting the stage for ·the evaluation. In the case of adults there are very few occasions that call for contacting the adults' place of work, even with their permission, to gather ancillary information about them. With children, however, relevant information obtained from their school and teachers would be extremely useful, if not crucial in many circumstances, though one is acutely aware that this is a sensitive issue in the Indian context, mainly because of the extremely close-knit nature of many Indian communities and subsequent concern about confidentiality issues in information gathering and exchange. The observation of and interaction with the younger child in play activities often provide information that is difficult to obtain otherwise, such as the activity and energy level of the child, capacity for sustained attention, preoccupations, and capacity for symbolic play to name a few. The attitude, stability or instability, personality functioning, awareness and related factors of the parents are extremely important in the evaluation and treatment of children, as most information and recommendations regarding the child have to be filtered through the parents. What information the parents may or may not reveal, what recommendations they will accept or reject (overtly or covertly) and related factors play a crucial role in evaluation and treatment.

In most child psychiatric evaluations one is dealing with three crucial variables: the child and the parents. At times there are other significant adults, such as grandparents or other extended family members who may bring in additional concerns and opinions that influence the evaluation. These are some of the ways in which the evaluation of children differ from that of adults.

An essential requirement in the child psychiatric evaluator is a genuine concern and empathy for the child and the parents. Parents and children are often in crisis by the time they are seen in an evaluation. They bring an array of concerns, anxieties, fears, hopes and despair. There is something unique about the problems and distress of children. In the parents' minds, childhood is the tender period of anticipation and hope for all good things to come. The very suspicion of development of psychiatric problems at such a tender age sets off an avalanche of emotions in all concerned. The evaluator who is not in tune with these unique concerns and turmoil often comes across as inept or crude in his dealings with the child and family, unaware of the distress and sensitivities of the people concerned. To obtain the confidence of the child in a genuine manner without making false or inappropriate promises is extremely important. Children often reveal information that is anxiety provoking, or embarrassing to them, if they feel that the evaluator will use the information in a sensitive manner to alleviate their problems. Adults will often settle for the technical expertise or reputation of a clinician. Not so with most children. They seldom 'open up' unless they feel they have in front of them a genuinely concerned, friendly and trustworthy ally.

At the outset it should be mentioned that there is no one set format for a good child psychiatric evaluation. A good knowledge of children's normal development and the possible manifestations of various psychiatric disorders at various developmental stages, in the cognitively well-endowed and the cognitively deficient child is an essential pre-requisite for conducting a good evaluation. Flexibility and capacity to improvise, depending on the needs of a given situation are the hallmarks of a good evaluator.

Psychiatric evaluation of the child is seldom complete without an informal evaluation of the parents also, with whom the child is intimately involved in a dependent relationship. This does not in any way imply that childhood psycho-pathology is caused by parental psychopathology. The relation-ship is far more subtle and complex. However, even if the problem arises primarily from within the child, the dependent intimate relation the child has with the family makes the expression of the problem often take an interpersonal colouring. The distress and or deviant behaviour in a child produces distress and or deviant behaviour in the parents and other family members, which would manifest in a multitude of ways depending on the vulnerabilities of the people concerned. Any treatment recommendation to be effective, would require the active cooperation of the parents, and without evaluating the personality structure, likes and dislikes of the parents, and the presence or absence of major psychopathology in them, one cannot make a treatment recommendation that would be accep-table and likely to succeed. This does not mean that the parents and other family members should be subjected to a formal psychiatric evaluation. How one approaches this issue is dis-cussed further in the 'Interviewing of the parents' section below.

Though at times children may have to be seen for the first time in an emergency visit, in general the evaluation should be a pre-arranged affair with the evaluator allotting enough of his or her undisturbed time for the evaluation of the child. On the average this would require about an hour-and-a-half of interview and observation time alone, even for an experienced clinician. Unless there is a need to implement pharmacological treatment or arrange for inpatient hospitalization immediately, it is best to complete the evaluation in two sessions, on separate days, perhaps a few days apart. This gives an opportunity to see the child on two separate occasions, enabling to observe how consistent or variable the child functioning is from time to time, and also providing a chance to observe the child free of some of the initial anxiety and inhibitions that are common when dealing with a stranger for the first time, and that too, in often stressful circumstances. It also helps in making a determination as to how transient, variable or persistent the presenting problem is. Another advantage in completing the evaluation in two visits is that, after the first visit, need for additional reports may become evident to complete a good evaluation, and this gives the parents time to make such reports available before the second visit, which will make the evaluation more thorough. Each session should end in a supportive manner without making false statements or raising false hopes. Often a child and parents would present in a busy outpatient setting having travelled considerable distance, hoping ·to be seen then and there and get started on a treatment course. It is only humane and proper that they be seen at least in a brief interview to assess the general nature of the problem, and the parents and child prepared for a more detailed evaluation at a later date, unless the situation calls for emergency or crisis intervention measures, in which case, it should be handled in such a manner by staff or emergency room personnel with training to address such situations, as spending enough unhurried time is crucial in the evaluation of children.

Children are not very forthcoming and information is often revealed in bits and pieces of relevant and not so relevant admixtures. Many a time their statements are vague, contradictory, or equivocal. One of the main reasons a child psychiatrist may succeed in doing good evaluations when others have failed, is because, he or she has been willing and able to spend enough time with the child and parents, gather and review additional information that may be obtainable to arrive upon well thought out conclusions. Rushing through a quick evaluation, except in an emergency, is unfair to the child, the family, as well as the evaluator herself. Once the need for adequate time is explained, most parents are willing to cooperate. In general once an evaluation is started, within a period of two weeks if not earlier, the evaluation should be completed and the parents and child (in a manner appropriate for the child) should be informed in lay terms what the evaluator thinks the nature of the problem is, and what measures may be helpful to alleviate the problem. In most cases detailed psychological tests and other relevant studies or consultations could be completed later.

It should be understood that the diagnostic understanding and formulation arrived upon after the evaluation is only preliminary and tentative. As the child is seen in treatment, and as further information and observations become available, some of the understandings may have to be modified as appropriate. In this sense the initial evaluation of the child has to be followed by a longitudinal evaluation that is ongoing as long as the child remains in treatment. Though this is pertinent for adults also it is more so for children, because of the rapid developmental process in children impacting on their problems, and because of the greater uncertainty involved in understanding and interpreting children's behaviour and symptomatology.

A child psychiatric evaluation should result in a well-written evaluation report. It is not only essential for present purposes, but for future references as well, sometimes even after the children reach adulthood.

Evaluation of children could be broadly divided into 5 sections

1. Interviewing the parents and obtaining relevant history and other information
2. Interview with child and observation of child in play activities (depending on age of child)
3. Medical-Neurological evaluation of the child, including obtaining appropriate laboratory tests, brain imaging studies, and specialists' consultations, as indicated
4. Evaluation of all data obtained, resulting in diagnosis and case formulation, and writing the evaluation report

5. Meeting with the parents (and child in an appropriate manner) in an informing session to explain the findings in lay terms and in an age appropriate and supportive manner, and the discussion of treatment options, if indicated

In most situations it is better to see the parents first, so that the evaluator could have a reasonable idea as to the general nature of the problem. An exception would be the case of an adolescent who specifically requests he or she be seen first either because of the belief that the parents would prejudice the mind of the interviewer by distorting information, or, because of frank suspiciousness.

### Interviewing the Parents

The parents are usually seen together. There are two main goals to accomplish during this interview. The first is to gather detailed information about the child's presenting problems, as well as, past history, family history, developmental history, school and social history and medical history. The second is an informal evaluation of parents as people and as parents of the child and parent's relationship with each other and the child. This is accomplished by observing the relevant processes as parents talk about the child, themselves, and by observing their interaction with each other and the child, and the emotional state and capacity for rational thinking the parents exhibit.

The interviewer should be sensitive to the feelings and concerns of the parents without sacrificing objectivity. The interview is conducted in a supportive manner, even though some parents may come across as defensive, argumentative, and even hostile. By the time a child is brought for psychiatric evaluation the parents would have been going through a mixture of feelings—anxiety, fear, depression, hopelessness, guilt and anger being the more common ones. Even the most seemingly unconcerned of parents would be blaming themselves in some way for having been responsible for the problems of the child. It is wise to keep a few things in mind when seeing the parents. The first and most important perhaps is that, in most instances of childhood psychopathology a complex combination and interaction of genetic—constitutional and environmental factors are at play, and to blame the parents as having been solely or even primarily responsible for the child's problems is naive if not dangerous in most cases. Parents should be viewed as having done what they could, given the totality of circumstances, which include among other things their own genetic make up and emotional vulnerabilities. Very little is accomplished by making the parents feel guiltier. Secondly, it is during the evaluation processs that the groundwork for positive therapeutic interventions and rapport are established, and the best of evaluations is of a little use unless it can be followed by helpful therapeutic intervention.

It is better to begin the interview by letting the parents elaborate with the minimum of interventions possible, the presenting problem, its development, course the problem has taken so far and related issues. At times it may be necessary to guide and re-focus the parents if they tend to become too circumstantial or scattered and irrelevant in their verbalizations for one reason or another. As the interview· proceeds, points and issues the interviewers feel are important could be brought up, explored and clarified in detail.

**The important areas to be covered in the interview with the parents include:**

1. Presenting problems and history of presenting problems. When and how did it/they manifest—the details of the various aspects and components of them—has it been improving, persisting without change, or, worsening? What interventions were tried, which ones helped and which did not? Ask about specific symptoms and signs that may be pertinent to the particular presenting problem. Ascertain if there was any likely precipitant.

2. Past psychiatric history and treatment history. Has the child had similar or other behavioural or emotional problems in the past? If so, what was done and what were the results? Enquire if the child has been fully well between the episodes or were there lingering or waxing and waning problems?

3. Developmental history. Start with the pre-natal history. Explore gently whether the pregnancy was expected or unexpected. How did the parents adjust to the pregnancy? What was the mother's/father's predominant emotional state

during pregnancy? Was the child born full term or premature? Was it a normal delivery, caesarean section or one that required another type of assistance? What was the birth weight? Any complications during labour, delivery or postnatal period? Did the child reach the usual developmental milestones at expected times or were they significantly delayed? Enquire specifically about when the child first rolled over, stood unassisted, and started walking. Enquire about the development of speech—when the child started saying the first words, phrases, sentences, whether the child was talkative or quiet to any unusual degree. Enquire whether there was any lag or arrest in speech development; if so what remedial measures were undertaken, if any, and what results occurred? Ask about the appearance of smiling, anticipatory posture, how the child responded to the parents' affectionate behaviour. Enquire when the child attained bowel and bladder control. Enquire about the child's early temperament. Was he or she easy to interact with child? Or did the child have a difficult temperament, difficult to please and manage, being extremely demanding, given to uncontrollable temper tantrums? Have such problems persisted or improved significantly? What was the child's sleep pattern during infancy, preschool years and later? Was the child underactive, normally active or hyperactive during infancy and later?

4. School and social history. Enquire how the child adjusted to the school on school entry. Was there persistent separation problem or school phobic behaviour? Was there significant behaviour/discipline problems in school? If so, how was it dealt with? Enquire about academic functioning in school-average, above average or significantly below average. If there are/were academic problems, were they present since early elementary school years, or did they start manifesting during adolescence only? Are there any indications of significant learning disabilities, and if there are, how was the problem dealt with? Enquire about the child's expectations for himself or herself regarding academics and future career choice and how they compare to the parental expectation for the child, and if there is a serious 'disparity between the two, how is the difference of opinion dealt with? Are the parents/ child, normally concerned or unconcerned, or overly

concerned and overanxious about examinations, marks, and such? Are studies over-emphasized in the home to the point that the other developmental needs of the child are neglected?

Enquire if the child is interested in and involved with his or her peers in the community.' Is the family socially involved or isolated? Ascertain if there are any problems of significant prejudices based on social status, religion, caste or colour that negatively impact the child one way or another. (Obviously explorations in these are as would take considerable tact and may or may not be much relevant in an individual child's situation.) Ascertain if the child is a victim of significant bullying or whether the child exhibits bullying behavior. In adolescence and older teens, it is important to keep in mind that the emerging sexuality and its vicissitudes would be crucial issues and the psychiatrist should have an open, knowledgeable, and unprejudiced attitude toward these aspects. In India, extreme prejudice toward homosexual and transgender individuals, places homosexual and transgender adolescents and youth in a worse predicament than in many, more enlightened parts of the world, even where the suffering of such youngsters is a well-known fact because of lingering prejudices.

An assessment should also be made of the general social skills or deficiencies of the child.

5. Parents' relationship to the child and parents' perception of the child's problems.

Ascertain if there is genuine affection and concern for this child from parents or guardians or do they appear to be mainly angry and hostile to the child. Do they have difficulty in expressing affection towards the child? Is the interaction with the child mostly in the form of criticisms of his or her performance or shortcomings? How is the child disciplined? Is there a history of harsh physical punishment or threats? (If there is, the parents should be advised in a supportive manner how important it is to refrain from such behaviour and how destructive such actions are for the child and their mutual relationship. Depending on the child protective laws of the particular locality, the clinician may have to initiate actions of informing the designated authorities if, it is suspected that a child is being abused or neglected). Determine if the child's relationship to the parents is based on mutual affection and concerns or is it mainly based on fear? Ascertain if the parents favour one or more among their children to the detriment of the child in question. If so, do they know why?

Enquire as to what the parents think is happening to their child and what kinds of measures they think could be helpful? Make a determination as to whether they see the child's problems as mainly 'bad behaviour' needing disciplinary measures only, or due to environmental stresses requiring environmental interventions, or to be addressed by advice, counselling or other psychotherapeutic measures only, or one that needs treatment with medicines. Enquire whether they are open to suggestions different from how they think the problem should be dealt with (this area of enquiry is very important in formulating a treatment plan that may be acceptable to the parents).

6. Family psychiatric history and family functioning.

This is arguably the most sensitive area in the interview with the parents. Enquire if any of the parents have a history of emotional / psychiatric problems identified and treated as such or not? If there is, what were the manifestations, the course of the problems, response to treatment? So also enquire if any of the siblings, grandparents, uncles and aunts have suffered from similar or related problems? Enquire about alcoholism and substance abuse among family members, and enquire also of the personality functioning of the alcoholic / substance abusing relative, if any. This is important because not only is there a tendency for alcoholism and other substance abuse to afflict all family members, but also many people suffering from affective illnesses, especially bipolar disorder, are often referred to by family members and others as having the problem of alcoholism only, with the manifestations of affective illness not recognized correctly because of the complicating alcohol or substance abuse, or because of the families' reluctance to acknowledge mental illness in one of their own, and also because many clinicians are not fully aware of such comorbidities. In this context it is important to note that, just because a parent or family member is identified as suffering from a particular psychiatric illness or problem, it does not mean that the child's problems are manifestations of the same illness or problem. In fact the child may be reacting to the stresses caused by illness of a parent or family member. However, with regard to one psychiatric illness, bipolar disorder, in a parent, grandparent or sibling, special attention should be given to determine if the child's serious behavioural or emotional problems are an early manifestation of this illness or its related variants, considering the high penetrance of this genetic illness in other family members and close relatives. Enquiry on such matters should be conducted in a very supportive and sensitive manner, as it provokes many concerns in the parents, but, is nevertheless an area that needs careful probing to complete a good evaluation. If the parents appear defensive and vague in their replies, do not persist on the enquiry to the point of breaking the rapport with them or making them very uncomfortable. With experience and an appreciation of the importance of this area of enquiry, one is able to elicit much valuable information and assess its relative importance in the child's problems.

Enquire about parents' own childhood, their families of origin, values their parents inculcated in them (and what values they inculcate in their children), their goals when growing up, their level of satisfaction or dissatisfaction with life, major reasons for unhappiness if any, parents' general philosophy of life, religious beliefs, how flexible or inflexible their belief systems are, superstitious beliefs, belief and practice of black-magic, witchcraft and such irrational ventures.

Assess how the parents get along with each other and how the child's problems impact on their relationship? Do they agree or disagree on how to deal with the child's problems? Are they blaming each other for the child's problems?

## Medical and Neurological History

Enquire if the child has any medical problems, acute or chronic. If the child does have significant medical problems, ascertain whether the psychiatric problems could be directly or indirectly related to it. Is there a history of hospitalizations of significance? Is there a history of prolonged anesthesia? Is there a history of seizure disorder? Make a determination as to how any medical/

neurological problem may be impacting on the child biologically and/or psychologically. It is important to know the medical status of the child not only in arriving at a proper diagnosis, but also in deciding on the nature of treatment measures, especially pharmacotherapy, which impacts on multiple systems.

### Interviewing the Child and Mental Status Examination

Ideally the child should be prepared for the interview in advance by the parents and/or referring person as to the nature of the visit. This, if properly done, will help minimize fear and negativism in the child.

In general, for interview purposes, children can be categorized into four, age or developmental groups: the preschool child, the elementary school-age child, the middle school or preadolescent child, and the adolescent/teenager.

Some general pointers regarding interviewing children are mentioned below.

Much has been written about the use of "play", especially its symbolic significance in the assessment and treatment *of* children in western countries. There is no doubt that play acts as a medium that allows for better observation and evaluation of the young child's spontaneous activity and verbalizations. However, the overemphasis on play as a diagnostic and therapeutic tool, especially the overemphasis on symbolic interpretation of play along psychoanalytic lines is of a little value in the Indian setting and elsewhere. This should, in no way, be construed as saying that play does not have a significant role in the evaluation and treatment of young children. It is useful to keep in mind a few points regarding the use of play in this context. Play serves the purpose of diffusing tension and putting the child at ease, so that anxiety laden topics could be probed gently as opportunities arise. Spontaneous and structured play also provide an additional and in some children a better opportunity than in a face to face interview, to assess the activity level, cognitive and representational (symbolic) capacity, capacity to concentrate, distractibility, impulsivity and capacity to follow adult directions among other things. Children provide glimpses of their style of dealing with the world during their play activities, and their spontaneous verbalizations during play give openings to the careful observer to further explore their concerns and conflicts. However, if not properly used, play could become hindrance in pursuing meaningful verbal interchange with the child in evaluation, and a form of avoidance in dealing with important issues in psychotherapy. It is the responsibility of the clinician to use the play time so that meaningful information may be obtained from the time spent and justify the expenses incurred by parents or third parties. Too often clinicians introduce the child into play activities with a little forethought as to the goals to be accomplished, and how to accomplish them leading to unproductive or chaotic sessions. Ideally the younger children are seen in a room that has at least a minimum amount of play materials that could be used for spontaneous and when necessary structured play. It is important to avoid having materials that could be used by an impulsive child in a dangerous or disruptive manner. A dollhouse with accompanying articles and figures, puppets representing family members, puzzles that can be put together without spending too much time, toy cars and trucks, simple two-person interaction board games, and parts that can be put together to make models, sets of crayons or pencils for drawing and colouring, and a supply of drawing and colouring papers, are often appropriate and adequate for most settings. A great deal of spontaneous play activity by the child could be observed even with minimal amounts of play material provided, if the child's interest is channeled skillfully by the interviewer.

All pre-school and early elementary school-age children should be given an opportunity to use play materials at least to some extent as part of the evaluation process. Much information could be obtained by providing a paper and pencil and asking the school age child to use it for writing and drawing and, copying geometrical figures. However, all children should be encouraged to take part in a direct verbal interchange that could be slowly guided towards the presenting problems and related issues without raising the discomfort level of the child too much. The pre-school child and the early elementary school-age child is best interviewed and observed through a combination of play and face to face interview, the middle-school-age child and the adolescent and older teen, mostly by direct interview, though paper and pencil tasks and activities are quite relevant and helpful in these age groups also.

In evaluating adults, usually the interviewer starts by asking what the presenting problem is. In the case of children, more often than not, this is to be avoided. The child is brought by others who have detected the need for a consultation. Even though, in most cases, the child is aware of this reason at least vaguely, often it is quite uncomfortable for the child to talk about it, especially to strangers. The early part of the evaluation should be spent· in making the child feel at ease and in developing rapport. This could be achieved in the younger child by either letting the child play, with the interviewer introducing a verbal interchange aimed at putting the child at ease and setting the tone for the interview, or by introducing and talking about neutral or pleasurable topics such as what kind of things they like to do, life at home and school, their friends, any interesting and pleasant things that happened recently, their family, their plans for the future, hobbies, television shows they like, areas in which they may have had creditable achievement, and such. As the interview progresses and rapport is established, there may be opportunities to bring up and explore issues related to the presenting problem and related concerns and conflicts. It is important to avoid raising the discomfort level of the child beyond a ·reasonable and tolerable level when exploring these issues. It would be helpful to keep in mind that the clinicians role is not that of a policeman or judge, but rather of one who tries to understand how the child may be feeling or behaving and why, or what may be making the child act one way or another, and what could be done to improve the situation.

A great deal of information is often obtained from younger children, if a playful quality is introduced into the interview, provided it is appropriate for the present mental state and circumstances of the child. In the interview of children, a great deal depends on the 'educated guess' the evaluator has about the child's problems. Rather than question the child, especially the younger child directly about such possibilities, it is often more fruitful to pose the questions in a hypothetical or indirect manner. For example, if the interviewer suspects that the anxiety generated because of her mother's and family's response to the diagnosis of a form of cancer in the mother, may be underlying the recent problematic separation anxiety and school phobia in a six year old child, rather than ask "are you afraid your mother is ·going to die? ", the interviewer may ask, while the child is engaged in doll play, "supposing there was this little girl and this mommy, and supposing the mommy was not feeling well and had to go to the hospital for check ups and operations and things like that, what will happen to the little girl you think? You think she'll be sad?, scared?, What kind of worries do you think she'll have?, Who can help her with these worries, you think? Who do you think can help her and look after her when the mommy is in the hospital?, When is the little girl going to be most worried and scared you think? What can she do not to be scared? Is there someone who can help her not to be too scared and upset?" and such questions in a tactful manner often can bring out leads that could be used in understanding the child's concerns that could be addressed in psychotherapy. Another technique is to acknowledge that the interviewer has seen many children go through the kind of turmoil the child may be experiencing in similar circumstances, and ask, if by chance he or she may be experiencing similar emotions. This may help the child elaborate on his inner feelings and concerns.

Some special but not uncommon situations in children require good preparation on the part of the clinician by gaining relevant experience in dealing with severely troubled children, under good supervision. For example, clinicians often are at a loss, as to how to approach a child who may be experiencing suicidal thoughts or auditory hallucinations. In a child who is suspected to be experiencing suicidal thoughts, one may enquire—"When you feel so bad or upset sometimes, do you feel like it is better not to be living? Or a thought comes to your mind that you want to die?". If the child acknowledges such thoughts or impulses, go on to gently explore how strong the thought or impulse may be. Explore in a calm and supportive manner "Does it bother you a lot?...., does it keep coming to your mind a lot, lot?,.... how does it make you feel?,....can you ignore it?...does it just go away quickly or will it keep on bothering you?" and such. If the child acknowledges intense suicidal thoughts, urges or death wishes, gently ask if he experiences these as thoughts or as his mind or someone else telling him to end his life. Any child who experiences strong suicidal thoughts or urges, of course, has to be further queried about any methods he or she feels like employing to end his or her life. Often children who are predisposed to experiencing intense emotionality when upset, report, on probing, a voice in their 'brain' or 'head' telling them to injure, kill themselves and such. So also, susceptible children, who frequently go into uncontrollable rages, fighting and generally exhibiting out of control behaviouur, which often give the appearance of 'bizarreness 'to their behaviour and actions when they are in such states, acknowledge on careful probing, an urging or voice in their 'head' or 'brain', that they may identify as their own or as the voice of another known or unknown person, urging them to 'fight', 'beat up 'others,' run around', 'be bad' and such. Children often report such phenomena, as occurring when they feel provoked by or angry at someone. These tendencies and phenomena go undetected in many severely troubled children because of the interviewer's inability to suspect such phenomena as occurring and skillfully probe to clarify the child's experiences. For most clinicians and others, such thoughts and experiences in a child are naturally unsettling, further interfering with their capacity to elicit such information and to arrive upon proper conclusions. A good deal of experience in dealing with severely troubled children, and a strong understanding of severe psycho-pathology in children are required to effectively evaluate and understand such problems in children.

There are some general areas to be covered during the Interview and mental status examination with the children, without being rigid about the format, but using them only as guidelines in a flexible manner depending on the given situation. It is important that the interviewer should get a 'sense' of what the child (especially the older child and adolescent) thinks of the reported presenting problems and related issues. As mentioned before this does not mean the interview should start with this topic. By the time the interview and observation sessions are concluded, one should have as good an understanding as possible, as to how the child experiences and understands the problems.

## Mental Status Examination

The mental status examination is the synthesis and interpretation of observations made throughout the interview with
the child. The following general areas should be covered as
part of the mental status examination in children.

### General Appearance and Behaviour

Observe the appearance of the child—does he look his age?
Appears physically healthy, or not? Are there obvious
dysmorphic features? Observe the attire and grooming. What
about the general demeanor of the child? His relatedness?; Is
he reasonably cooperative? Unusually fearful or shy? Are there
any striking separation problems from the parents, much more
than what one would expect from a child of his or her age?

Note that most children come across as somewhat inhibited
during the initial interview. Lack of such normal inhibition in
the form of intrusive behaviour, impulsivity, and over-
talkativeness often give the first clue as to likely emotional/
behavioural dyscontrol problems. So also, signs of significant
developmental delays or disorders are often evident within a
short time of meeting the child, from his or her appearance,
general behaviour, speech or lack of it, and manner of relating.
(However, one should keep in mind also that a developmentally
disordered child is, as, or more prone, than a cognitively well-
endowed child, to have additional psychiatric problems.)

Note the activity level of the child. Is he or she normally
active, underactive or overactive? What about impulsivity?
'Note also that, many hyperactive and impulsive children will
not exhibit these features in a significant manner when seen in
one to one interview with an adult authority figure who is a
stranger to them. Observations during spontaneous play and,
while in the waiting area, with other children or siblings, in
less restrictive settings, and in the class room would be more
revealing about this aspect of the child's functioning. This is
one of the reasons why teacher reports are extremely useful in
identifying such problems, especially when there is great
disparity between what is reported by the parents and what
the clinician observes in the initial interview. In this context

one should also keep in mind that what one observes in a clinical interview is at best only an approximation of the child's behaviour in his 'natural environment'. Just because a child appears not very hyperactive or impulsive when seen in the clinician's office, one should not disbelieve the parents' or teachers' report that the child is very hyperactive and impulsive. However, if one has not been able to verify such behaviour by direct observation one should suspend a final opinion on the matter, until further observations and information from other sources become available.

Observe also whether the child appears well coordinated in his or her movements or actions or if there are indications of a poorly coordinated neuromuscular system. Such observations give indication as to whether a more detailed neurological evaluation may be indicated.

### Intelligence

Make a general estimate of the child's cognitive functioning from the manner in which the child conducts himself or herself, the general knowledge the child exhibits, the social awareness or lack of it exhibited, the child's capacity for self-care and the academic capacities the child possesses in the case of the school age child. If there are obvious concerns about the child's cognitive capacities, the child may have to be referred for standardized assessment of cognitive and related capacities and functioning, if it has not been done already or get the reports if they have been done before coming to a final conclusion as to the nature of the child's problems.

### Speech and Language Development

Observe the level of speech and language development. Are there obvious, significant, problems in articulation, fluency of speech, the level of vocabulary the child has, and receptive and expressive language capacities? Is there evidence· for distorted or deviant language use indicative of a formal thought disorder? Is the child echolalic beyond what is expected for his or her age, which, most often points to a significant developmental disorder? Note also, if the child exhibits particular preoccupations or mixing up of fantasy and reality beyond what is expected for his age. Make a special note whether the child appears over-talkative, or his expressions show a lack of normal inhibitions.Though over-talkativeness could be a normal variation, it is also often a strong indicator of emerging mood disorders when accompanied by other related pathological problems.

## Mood and Affect

Observe the general mood of the child, and the affective range and variations. Is the child depressed? Irritable? If so, assess the intensity of these. Observe for additional features of depression and other mood disorders such as affective lability, pathological excitability, and euphoria. In younger children, separating from parents would be often a major problem in the interview setting, complicating the assessment of mood and affect of the child. Observe the level of anxiety and fear they exhibit when separating, and also whether the anxiety diminishes appropriately with reassurance and encouragement from the parents and the clinician. If it becomes very difficult for the child to separate from the parents, do not insist on it to an unreasonable degree. Many younger children, especially of pre-school age, may have to be interviewed in the parents' presence, because of separation problems. However, an attempt should be made to see the child with and without the parent or parents to elicit a more comprehensive understanding of the child, though this may not be possible in some younger children. The evaluator has to develop skills as to how to conduct the interview of the child with and without the parents.

## Thought Processes

Determine if the thought processes are properly connected and goal oriented (it takes considerable experience to make this determination in younger children who normally talk in a somewhat disjointed manner and in incomplete sentences and phrases). Is there evidence for a formal 'thought disorder'? (One should not mistake expressive language disorder such as one sees in developmentally disordered children for formal thought disorder, which is a rare phenomenon in children). Does the child show pressured speech with sudden and frequent shifting from topic to topic? Does the child's thinking appear difficult to follow because of intermixing of fantasy or delusions and reality? (note, that it will take considerable experience and repeated observations often, to make such determination in younger children). It is better to reserve judgement when one is uncertain on such matters, rather than hastily conclude that a child is experiencing psychotic phenomena or cannot distinguish fantasy and reality.

### Fantasy Life and Dreams

Getting a sense of the child's longings and desires, even the imaginary scenarios that all children entertain from time to time give a sense of the child's inner life.

Ask what he or she wants to be in the future and what are the plans or methods to accomplish it?. Asking the child what he or she would choose, given three magic wishes, is a time honoured and useful avenue to gain inroads into the wishes and preoccupations of children, without directly pressing them to reveal their inner desires. Most children who are not significantly distressed about one thing or another, will wish for a combination of material things that children in their particular culture value, at times along with a wish to be famous and rich, for success in studies, future career, these at times combined with good things to happen for their family members. Children, who have particular preoccupations or worries often give glimpses of their concerns when answering this question. The very manner in which they approach this question itself can be highly revealing. Children who are depressed or highly distressed about one thing or another often have difficulty even coming up with any three wishes. Some children who are very unhappy because of separation from or loss of a parent state just one wish: To be with the parent from whom they are separated, or for the parent who died to be alive again. Enquiring about any dreams of a repetitive nature or theme could also be revealing about concerns, wishes and fears the children may have.

### Play

Observe the interest children show in play and play materials. Note how impulsive or not they may be in their approach to play and play materials. Observe whether the play is organized or chaotic. Pay attention to their spontaneous verbalizations during play. Note especially, the appropriate or inappropriate use of play materials, including use of materials that represent an object in an appropriate manner (representational or symbolic play). This is especially important in the evaluation of children who are cognitively' impaired or suspected to be suffering from a pervasive developmental disorder such an autistic disorder, in whom such representational or symbolic use of objects will be deficient.

A simple two-person board game such as checkers, that have a competitive aspect, helps demonstrate a child's capacity to take part in a meaningful interaction with another, to remain focused and goal directed, his or her capacity for frustration tolerance, a sense of the child's cognitive capacities and, reaction to winning or losing among other strengths or weaknesses. One has to be careful not to spend too much time in play during the interview, however, as some children would have difficulty disengaging from play once they are introduced to it and one may end up not having sufficient time for direct 1:1 interview away from the play setting.

### Special Symptoms

Enquire and observe for symptoms or phenomena such as obsessions, compulsions, phobias, hallucinations or delusions, or anything that stands out as unusual about the child's utterances or behaviour. If one is unsure of a particular behaviour that appears unusual, gently ask the child if he can explain what prompts the behaviour or what it means.

### Child's Awareness of his or her Problems

Make a determination as to whether the child has a general awareness as to the nature of his or her problems. Does he believe that he has a problem that requires help—from others who deal with such problems?, or does he think that he has no problems and that the parents and others are exaggerating or making false statements? Does he think that he is merely responding to the problems actually caused by others? and that they are the people who really need help in changing their behaviour? Determine if the child appears amenable to suggested interventions, when the nature of the problem and the possible interventions that could be helpful are explained to him or her.

To cover all the areas mentioned above will obviously take considerable amount of time and effort and cooperation from the child. Not all areas, however, need to be covered in detail with all children. The clinician should use his intuition and experience to decide which are as should be concentrated upon as the interview progresses.

### Medical-neurological Examination and Laboratory Studies

Psychiatric examination of the child is never complete without a good medical-neurological examination, including baseline laboratory studies. Whether the evaluating clinician should do the screening medical-neurological evaluation depends on the individual situation and the clinician. The important point is that the evaluating physician should feel comfortable that he or she is well aware of the medical-neurological status of the child. With most children who are under regular follow up from their pediatrician, are sent report from the doctor should provide most of the information that is necessary, to be supplemented by additional consultations, imaging studies, as the psychiatrist may consider relevant. Children in whom neurological or contributory medical problems are suspected should of course be referred to the relevant specialists for further studies.

### Evaluation and Synthesis of all Available Data, Diagnosis, and Formulation

Once the interview and examinations are completed, the clinician should gather and review all the information obtained including any school reports, psychological test reports, medical consultation reports, and laboratory reports that may be available. This should result in the clinician having a good understanding of the child and his problems in the bio-psychosocial sense, which should lead to a comprehensive formulation of the total situation, and diagnoses using the standard accepted nomenclature.

The formulation or case formulation is essentially a summary statement of the clinician's understanding of the child and his problems—how the child came to be what he or she is, what the problems are and how they came to be. Considerationis given to all the-factors: Genetic-constitutional, family, environmental, and intra-psychic. Not only the deficiencies but also the strengths of the child should be mentioned, because, often it is on the strengths that one is able to build a recovery and habilitation or rehabilitation. Each factor is weighed according to the major or minor role it plays, in the production and maintenance of the problem. As more information becomes available in the future, the formulation may have to be modified as appropriate.

Making formal diagnoses according to internationally accepted nomenclature and criteria is important, keeping in mind, however, the limitations involved. Diagnoses in child psychiatry is even more fluid and uncertain than in adult psychiatry where it remains mostly at an empirical, uncertain state. However, without formally diagnosing the problem it is difficult to formulate an appropriate treatment plan and communicate effectively with other professionals involved, as to the general nature of the problem. It is important to know where the child's problems anchor—whether one is seeing most likely a transient reaction to a stressor, or the manifestation of a more genetic, constitutionally based mental illness that may run a more protracted course. Also, the substantially different ways in which these problems have to be addressed calls for as reasonable a diagnostic understanding as one can arrive upon. In addition progress in the field as a whole depends on clinicians making as accurate a diagnosis as possible, and correcting it with treatment measures indicated for it and determining what works and what does not, and to understand how much of what types of problems exist in the community, so that, scarce resources, both in treatment and research, could be allocated in the most appropriate manner.

### Meeting with Parents and Child in the Informing Session

Once the clinician has come to a preliminary conclusion, he should meet with the parents (and if a team is involved in the evaluation and treatment, they also), and in lay terms explain to them in a supportive manner what the understandings are about the child and his problems and what measures may be helpful. Depending on the age and the capacity of the child to understand helpful information, the nature of the problem and measures that a resuggested to bring about improvement should be explained in a comforting and supportive manner to the child also in a language that a child of his or her developmental level can understand. It is better to see the parents alone first to discuss the findings and recommendations in a detailed manner and then have the child join the session so information that the child can understand and will not be too upsetting for him or her could be discussed in an appropriate manner. Information that is of very little therapeutic value and that could cause undue distress to the people concerned should not be divulged. The parents and child should be given an opportunity to ask any questions they may have about the feedback given to them and the measures suggested.

## THE CHILD PSYCHIATRIC EVALUATION REPORT

The evaluation should result in a well written Child Psychiatric Evaluation Report, documenting the problems, findings and recommendations. This may take at least a half-an-hour in most cases. This report should preferably be typed, so it will be legible, as it may be of use for years to come as many clinicians who may come across the same child in the future would find a good evaluation report from the past of great assistance. Nowadays, in the United States, the psychiatrist produces the report on the computer either during the evaluation interview or immediately following it and this saves time, but writing the report during the interview itself has its advantages and disadvantages. Also, nowadays there is a trend in the United States to use a standard evaluation form with yes or no answers to be checked off to the questions about the child. Though this saves time, many of these types of reports fail to convey a really useful sense of the child and his or her problems and is certainly much inferior to a well-written evaluation report by the psychiatrist.

**The report should contain the following elements:**

Identifying data and date of evaluation

Presenting problems (according to parents and other concerned adults, and according to the child)

History of presenting problems and past history

Developmental history

School and social history

Family functioning and family psychiatric history

Medical neurological history and significant findings

Include a brief description of interview with the child (including description of the child and his or her general behaviour, pertinent observations from the child's play and 1:1 interview / interactions, and quotes from the child that may be highly revealing of the child and his problems and would give the reader a 'vivid picture' of the child—especially the type of information that cannot be conveyed by a mental status examination. The child's response to 'three magic wishes' could also be included in this section.

**Mental Status**

General description of the child—appearance, general behaviour, activity level, impulsivity

Cooperativeness Relatedness

Cognitive functioning

Speech and language capacities

Mood and affect (and suicidal risk if pertinent) Presence or absence of formal thought disorder and related phenomena

Special symptoms (significant tics, motor abnormalities, obsessions, compulsions, phobias, hallucinations, delusions)

Child's awareness/understanding of his/her problems (insight)

Formulation (a short paragraph as to the nature of the problem, contributing factors, and how the present situation came about without being too speculative or theoretical).

# Examination of the Elderly Patients

S Kalayanasundaram,   R Johnson   Pradeep

*"Old age is not a disease—it is strength and survivorship, triumph over all kinds of vicissitudes and disappointments, trials and illnesses"*

Maggie Kuhn

## INTRODUCTION

"Elderly" have been defined as a person who is 65 years or greater according to WHO. However, there is no consensus whether the cut off should be 60 or 65 years in some countries. Currently, elderly are classified as young old (65–74 years), old (75–84 years), oldest old (over 85 years) and frail elderly (anyone over 65 years with physical and/or cognitive infirmity) (Hobbs and Damon, B, 1996). India has ranked as the second most populous country in the world and has 102 million people (> 60 yrs) as estimated in the year 2011. India's increasing life expectancy and decreasing fertility rate has led to the rapid increase in the elderly population, resulting in WHO terming it as the 'Ageing' Country. This has resulted in increased burden on the resources and high dependency ratio. Due to the physiological and cognitive changes, the elderly are vulnerable to both communicable and non-communicable diseases. In India, the Elderly or Geriatric Healthcare is still in the nascent stage of development and needs to grow. There is a dire need to have a National Policy for the care of the elderly.

In this chapter, we would be covering very important points for postgraduates and clinicians to consider while taking a detailed history and conducting a physical and mental state

155

examination. Then we would be giving a brief review of all the important standardized interviews and rating scales available currently to assess cognitive functions, depression and caregiver's burden in the elderly. Later, a review of important lab investigations (routine and specialized tests) and neuroimaging which needs to be considered in the management of the elderly patients are tabulated. Then the chapter would discuss about the latest updates on important psychosocial issues. We also have briefly covered some important topics such as organic conditions (delirium, mild cognitive impairment and dementia), depression and psychotic disorders in the elderly. In the end, we have constructed tables to differentiate between delirium vs dementia and pseudodementia vs dementia.

## HISTORY-TAKING AND MENTAL STATE EXAMINATION IN THE ELDERLY

### HISTORY-TAKING

History-taking is a very important skill in psychiatry. It is an art which have to be learnt through active listening, eliciting symptoms, interviewing appropriately and observing during the interview. It provides vital information in the diagnostic work-up of a patient. There are certain difficulties which can be encountered with the elderly which includes emergence of new symptoms and having preconceived ideas about their disorders, they may forget a few important details in history and may have severe cognitive deficits or may give too many details and also possibly exaggerate their symptoms. Hence, the psychiatrist should have the patience to get the information and should not try to hurry up the interview. They may require at least two to three interviews to collect the history and also to collect information from their relatives also. Here we are attempting to give some valuable tips to focus and derive information from the elderly persons.

### PRESENTING COMPLAINTS

- Elderly persons may have sensory deficits which may affect the history-taking, hence it is important in the beginning of the interview to ask them for any sensory problems and provide appropriate help.

- It may be required to talk to them slowly and clearly.
- They may under report symptoms or present with non-specific symptoms such as vague pains or may amplify their distress.
- They may have mild to severe cognitive deficits, hence information has to be corroborated with a reliable family member or relative or an attender.
- It is also important to know the elderly persons attitude and level of comfort with the family members or care-takers.
- It should also focus on functional abilities (activities of daily living), behavioural issues and social interactions.
- Substance abuse should be asked for in elderly who have past history of substance use. Sometimes elderly patients continue to take medications prescribed by their physicians such as benzodiazepine and can become dependent on the same.
- Current social settings such as current living arrangement (own house, relative's house or old age homes), the primary care-taker, support systems (religious services or spiritual services) of the elderly should be elicited.
- A brief review about how the situation of the house will give a lot of clues to the diagnosis. Dirty, unclean houses and locked window could point to a psychotic or depressive disorder.
- Negative history such as organic mental disorders, substance use, psychotic disorders, mood disorders, anxiety and somatoform disorders should be excluded.

## PAST PSYCHIATRIC AND MEDICAL HISTORY

- Information about the past psychiatric and medical histories (including current medical problems and the medications they are consuming) are very helpful for current management and follow-up.
- Information about past pharmacological, surgical and non-pharmacological treatments is very important for the future planning. It is important to ask about the dosage, duration, effectiveness and side-effects of previous medications.

## FAMILY HISTORY

- A three generation pedigree chart may be useful. For each member a detailed account of their age, educational level, relationship with the proband, similar diagnosis if any, the age of onset of that disorder and what medications have helped them with a particular disorder; may help in the diagnosis and treatment of the patient.
- Family history should focus on genetic disorders (Alzheimer's disease, Huntington's disease, certain neuromuscular disorders, diabetes, hypertension) or inherited disorders.

## OCCUPATIONAL HISTORY

- Educational level attained, trainings received and details about the previous jobs (such as part-time or full time, promotions, issues with employer, job satisfaction) and the current employment should be documented.

## NUTRITIONAL ASSESSMENT

- It is a vital part of history taking; since they are at a greater risk of vitamin and mineral deficiencies. Some of the common deficiencies found in them include vitamins A, $B_{12}$, C, D, calcium, sodium, iron and zinc.
- A brief method of looking for any nutritional deficiencies include brief nutritional history using the Nutritional Health Checklist, then a 24-hr recall of the food intake, then to do a physical examination to look for signs of malnutrition, inadequate vitamins or minerals and to do selected lab tests to detect for nutritional deficiencies based on history and examination.

## PHYSICAL EXAMINATION

In the OPD, priority should be given to the elderly patients because they may not be able to sit for a long time, have difficulty standing for a long time, sitting on wheelchair may be discomforting, may be anxious or restless due to psychiatric conditions. Adequate time to enter and exit the consultation room should be given to prevent any falls or injuries. They also usually prefer a family member or a relative to be present during the interview; sometimes they may want to speak about confidential issues, then their privacy should be respected.

## GENERAL EXAMINATION

Look for the body built, nutrition and any weight loss (tuberculosis, HIV or depression) as per family's observation and history.

Examination of the thyroid, pallor, icterus, edema and the skin (erythema, ulceration, premalignant or malignant lesions) may give clues to major disorders.

### Vital Signs

There may be difficulties in assessing the vital signs but care must be taken to do the procedures slowly and with less discomfort to the elderly.

Pulse should be assessed in the wrist, neck, abdomen, groin and feet. Blood pressure should be checked in both the arms and preferably in the resting state. Orthostatic hypotension has to be checked in them since it is very common and sometimes induced by some of the medicines they are taking for other medical conditions. There can be an overestimation of the blood pressure in the elderly due to stiffness of the arteries and have to be cautious when giving antihypertensives to them.

Fundus examination should always be done and it can give vital information about bleeds, retinal tears or raised intra-cranial pressures.

### Head

Look for facial weakness (stroke or transient ischaemic attacks), temporal artery swelling or tenderness (giant cell arteritis and polymyalgia rheumatic) and frontal bossing (Paget's disease).

In the eyes look for cataract, impaired vision, bleeds, loss of central vision (age-related macular degeneration) and loss of peripheral vision (glaucoma).

In the ears, assess for hearing loss due to foreign body impaction, ear wax, acoustic neuroma, faulty hearing aid or its placement and Paget's disease.

In the neck look for carotid bruits (Aortic stenosis, cerebrovascular disease) and thyroid enlargement (hypothyroidism or hyperthyroidism). It is also important to look for the flexibility of the neck. If there is any difficulty or resistance to passive flexion, extension, and lateral rotation, then a cervical spine disorder should be suspected but if there is resistance to flexion and extension, then meningitis should be suspected.

The mouth should be examined for bleeding or swollen gums, loose or broken teeth, fungal infections, and signs of cancer (e.g. leukoplakia, erythroplakia, ulceration or mass).

## Neurology

A detailed examination of the sensory and motor system is required. It is important to look for tremors of extremities (Parkinson's disease, drug induced EPS), muscle wasting (atrophy, stroke), gait disturbances (Parkinson's disease, foot deformities, arthritis, stroke) and sensory loss (vitamin deficiencies).

## Breasts

Examination of the breast should be assessed in both genders. In women, always remember to have a chaperone to avoid sexual abuse. It is important to examine for any masses such as fibroadenoma and cancer.

## Chest

To look for barrel chest (emphysema), kyphosis, scoliosis and shortness of breath (chronic obstructive pulmonary disease, bronchial asthma, cardiomyopathy, congestive heart failure).

In the cardiac examination, look for fourth heart sound (S4) (left ventricular thickening) and systolic ejection, regurgitant murmurs. The murmurs of aortic stenosis, aortic insufficiency and mitral regurgitation (valvular arteriosclerosis) should not be missed.

During the auscultation of the lungs, check by any abnormal breath sounds or irregular air entry.

## Abdomen

Examination for surgical scars, organomegaly, pulsatile masses (aortic aneurysm) or any other masses should be attempted.

## GENITO-URINARY

In both the genders, attempt should be made to identify any faecal incontinence (faecal impaction, rectal cancer, rectal prolapse), urinary incontinence (bladder or uterine prolapse, detrusor instability, estrogen deficiency) or rectal mass (colorectal cancer).

In the males, prostate enlargement (benign prostatic hypertrophy) or nodules (prostate cancer) should be specifically looked for and not missed.

In the females, to look for atrophy of the vaginal mucosa due to estrogen deficiency and cervical masses (cervical cancer).

## MENTAL STATE EXAMINATION

### General Appearance

It is important to look at the grooming (ill-kempt in depressed, dishevelled in psychotic patients or increased in hypomanic or manic), personal hygiene (may be poor in depressed or psychotic) and dressing (inappropriate or poor matching of clothes or clothes may have been put on in the wrong order may be seen in elderly with cognitive dysfunction). Establishing rapport with the elderly is very important.

### Psychomotor activity (PMA)

Reduced PMA is found in elderly with delirium, catatonic symptoms, major depression and severe psychotic symptoms. Increased PMA is found in severe anxiety, mania, agitated depression and dementia (moderate to severe). Any abnormal movements such as tics, tardive dyskinesia (dystonia, akathisia and EPS), dystonia or tremors have to be recorded.

### Affect

Facial expression may be limited and a full range of emotional expressions may not be seen in the elderly as compared to younger patients. Flat or blunted affect may be found in psychotic patients.

## Thought

It is very important to know whether the elderly person is able to hear and reciprocate to your questions. Sometimes they may have hearing problems or dysphasia (expressive, receptive or global); which should not be mistaken for formal thought disorder (FTD). FTD are not as common in the elderly when compared to the younger population.

Slowed flight of ideas is seen in the elderly manic patient and it can be easily missed.

Preoccupations of health problems, phobias, obsessions, compulsions, hypochondriacal beliefs, somatic symptoms, depressive cognitions are very common presentation in the elderly.

Depressive cognitions such as worthlessness, hopelessness and helplessness can be present in the depressed elderly and they have high risk for suicidal attempt. Suicidal ideas and homicidal ideas should be elicited.

Nihilistic delusions, delusional parasitosis, partition delusions and delusions of stealing of property are very common psychotic symptoms in the elderly.

## Perceptions

Illusions and hallucinations may not be very prominent in the elderly and may be only transient due to reduced sensory acuity.

## Cognitive functions

### Orientation

This is a vital assessment for elderly patients. Traditionally, it does not come first in the cognitive functions. However, in the elderly; disorientation is common and a lot of time can be wasted if it is not assessed in the beginning. Typically, the orientation is assessed in four areas; they include time (time, day, date, month, year and season), place (ward, building and floor), the person (self and others) and the situation (where are they now and what is their current situation). It is important to know that time moves faster than the place, person and situation and hence it is the first to be lost in confused or disoriented person.

**Attention and concentration:** The attention is assessed by the Digit Span Test and the concentration is assessed by 'A' Random Letter Test and Serial Subtraction Test.

**Digit Span Test:** It is conducted by asking a patient to repeat a series of digits read to him by the examiner with one second duration without repetition and should not be grouped. Patients should first be tested on retention of digits forward (maximum possible) and then in reverse order (maximum possible). If the patient has understood the test and fails the test twice, then the test should be stopped and attempted later. The average expected level for elderly 65 to 74 yrs, with an education level of 10th standard for digit span forward test is 7.6 (+ 2.5) in males and 6.7 (+ 2) in women and for the digit span backward test it is 5.4 (+ 1.5) in males and 5 (+1.5) in females.

**'A' Random Letter Test:** It is a simple test of concentration where the subjects are asked to indicate the letter A whenever it is being read out with a long series of random alphabets.

**Serial Subtraction Test:** It is important to first know whether the person has a formal education and they do not have poor arithmetic skills. The subject is asked to subtract one from 20, count backwards and stop at zero. Make sure that they have understood the test. Once the test has started, note the total time taken to complete and the number of errors made. There are alternative tests such as subtraction of 3 from 40; months of the year, days of the week—forward and backward can also be asked.

## Memory

The examiner needs to assess all the aspects of memory. This will help in differentiating the type of memory loss, the degree of memory loss and the impact of the memory deficit on the patient's ability to function. The tests of memory include immediate memory, recent memory, recent verbal memory, recent visual memory and remote memory.

**a. Immediate memory** is tested by digit span test.

b. **Recent memory** (new learning ability): It is the ability to remember information from minutes, hours, or days ago. Usually interviewers assess for recall of the events of last 24 – 48 hrs and by corroborating it from a reliable informant. It is important to know the temporal sequencing of the events, any confabulation or false memories in the retrieval, any selective loss of memory about any special incident or theme. In the case of patients with head injury, particular attention needs to be paid to any anterograde or retrograde amnesia. Elderly in the age group of 60 to 70 years can recall 13 to 15 facts.

c. **Recent verbal memory**: It is tested by the interviewer introduces himself with his name or house address and then requests the patient to repeat his name to ensure that he has registered it. After 5 minutes, he asks the patient to repeat his name. A patient with memory problems may deny that he heard your name or may not be able to recall. If he fails to recall for three times it is suggestive of recent verbal memory impairment. It is important to remember that there is no hearing loss in the patient before you begin the test.

d. **Recent visual memory**: It is tested by presenting 3 to 5 unrelated objects by the interviewer and asked to name all of these. Then he should hide the objects in different places while allowing the patient to watch. Distract the patient by talking to him and after 5 minutes ask the patient to tell and take out the objects from their respective places. Less than 3 recalls is abnormal. It is important to rule out any nominal aphasia and visual agnosia.

e. **Remote memory**: It is the ability to remember things that happened years ago.

   a. Personal events: It is tested by asking the patient about their birthday, anniversary day, the first time he met his wife and the first child's name.

   b. Impersonal events: Some important political or public events in his life can be elicited.

In the early phase of Alzheimer's dementia, the remote memory may be intact but the recent and immediate memory can be affected.

## Intelligence

Intelligence is defined in different ways and to simply describe "it is a process that involves the understanding of complex ideas, adapting effectively to the environment and the capacity of the person to use the resources more effectively to complete a given task".

The bedside assessment of the intelligence involves tests on language, comprehension, abstraction, judgement, general information and calculation. Before you begin the cognitive assessment you need to assess whether the patient is right or left-handed. This will give us information about which is the dominant and non-dominant side of the brain. Standard test can be used to assess the Intelligence quotient (IQ).

a. **Language functions:** Language is an important component of the cognitive functions. It is the only way we can understand what a person is thinking and planning. Some of the aspects of language which needs to be assessed are articulation, fluency, comprehension, repetition, naming, word finding, reading, writing and prosody.

b. **General fund of information:** Before you begin the test, it is important to know the subject's educational status and socio-occupational background.

For subjects with formal education:

• Name five PMs of India.

• Name five rivers of India.

• Name five capital cities of India.

For subjects without formal education or from rural background:

• Seasons?

• Prices of food?

• Prices of land?

• What crops are grown at a particular season?

c. **Comprehension:** It is the ability of a person to understand, process the information and respond to the questions relevantly.

- What will you do when you feel cold?
- What will you do if it rains when you start to work?
- What will you do when you miss a bus when you are on a journey?

d. **Arithmetic:** It is important to assess whether the person is able to understand the basic arithmetic like addition, subtraction, division and multiplication. Then an attempt should be made to five simple problem based calculation and increase the severity of the calculation.

- How much is 4 rupees and 5 rupees?
- I borrowed 6 rupees from a friend and returned 2 rupees. How much do I still owe to him?
- If 18 boys are divided into 6 groups, how many groups will there be?

e. Vocabulary is assessed by looking the range of use of simple to complex words and their meanings during the interview.

f. **Abstract ability:** Abstraction is the process of taking away or removing characteristics from something in order to reduce it to a set of essential characteristics. In simple terms, it is the ability to shift back and forth between general concepts and specific examples. This is tested by *proverb interpretation and test of similarity and dissimilarity*.

    i. **Proverb interpretation:** It is a used to assess verbal abstractions. The examiner looks for the ability of the patient to understand the metaphor and then to generalized intended meaning of the proverbs. The patient is first inquired whether he knows any proverbs used by his relatives. If yes, then he is asked to report and ask the both literal and metaphorical meaning of same. The interpretation may be concrete, semiabstract or abstract. Poor abstraction may occur in schizophrenia, dementia or subnormal intelligence.

    Given below is an example of various responses to a proverb.

    "All that glitters is not gold" is an old proverb. It speaks of individuals who just boast but do nothing in action. This response would be graded as abstract response.

    In semi-abstract response the patient may partially interpret the proverb in an abstract way but has not understood it fully.

In concrete response the patient would just repeat the proverb or put it in different words and not the actual inner meaning of the proverb.

**Proverbs for interpretation:**

1. Don't count your chickens before they are hatched.
2. There is no use crying over spilt milk.
3. A stitch in time saves nine.

  ii. **Test of similarity and dissimilarity** between two overtly dissimilar situations, which requires analysis of relationships formation of verbal concepts and logical thinking.

### Similarities Test

Here, two items are given and the patients are asked what is similar between the two items. Expected answers are given in the bracket.

a. Apple    — Orange (Fruits)
b. Tiger    — Cat (Animals)
c. Nose     — Ear (Sense organs)

Differences: Similarly, differences between two objects can also be asked.

a. Stone    — Potato (non-edible/ edible)
b. TV       — Radio (Visual/ audio)
c. Praise   — Punishment (Positive/negative)

**Judgement:** It refers to the person's capacity to make sound, reasoned and responsible decisions. Generally, hypothetical questions about how a patient has responded or would respond to real-life challenges. It assesses the patient's executive system capacity; in terms of impulsiveness, social cognition, self-awareness and planning ability. If it is impaired due to mental illness, it has implications for his own safety and others.

**There are three types of judgement:**

  i. Social: This is inferred from historical information and observation of behaviour in the ward (vide social manner).
 ii. Personal: Personal logic about present and future—how do you explain the present state, what is your plan for the future?

iii. Test: Responses in test situations, a letter on the road, house on fire, this component has poor validity.

### Insight

The capacity to recognize that one has an illness that requires treatment is called insight (Ghaemi, 1997). The three important components to assess insight are: Awareness (recognition that one has a mental illness), attribution (ability to re-label unusual mental events (such as delusions and hallucinations) as pathological) and adherence (willingness to take treatment).

**Diagnosis:** Based on the above assessment a diagnostic formulation can be attempted and a provisional diagnosis can be made. A three axial diagnosis of ICD-10 or 5 axial diagnosis of DSM-IV can be used.

### STANDARDIZED INTERVIEWS AND RATING SCALE IN THE ELDERLY

1. Cognitive dysfunction scales
   A. Delirium assessments scales
      i. Screening scales
      ii. Diagnostic scales
   B. Dementia assessments scales
      i. Screening/shorter scales
      ii. Longer scales
      iii. Activities of daily living (ADL) scales
      iv. Behaviour
      v. Quality of life scales
2. Depression rating scales
3. Carer burden scale

### COGNITIVE DYSFUNCTION SCALES

### Delirium Assessments Scales

#### Screening Scales

There are many scales used for the screening of delirium depending on the ward, settings and personnel. They include NEECHAM confusion scale, nursing delirium screening scale, delirium observation screening scale/delirium observation scale (DOS), intensive care delirium screening checklist and global attentiveness rating. It has been found that the most suitable instrument for screening patients in surgical and general medical wards includes NEECHAM confusion scale and DOS; CAM-ICU was better in ICU settings.

NEECHAM confusion scale has a 3 subscales (9 items) and takes only 10 mins to administer. It has a very good inter-rater reliability, good validity and high sensitivity and specificity. It is used by the nurses in different situations such as nursing homes, medical wards and ICUs. It has a total score of 30, a score of 27–30 indicates normal functioning, 25 and 26 suggests "not delirious" but at high risk, 20 to 24 suggests mild and a score below 20 points indicates moderate to severe delirium.

Delirium Observation Scale (DOS) is a dichotomously scored and 13-items scale derived from the delirium observation screening scale. It is scored by taking an average of 3 shifts by a nursing staff and a score greater than 3 suggests delirium.

### Diagnostic Scales

The commonly used scales for diagnostic assessment of delirium include delirium symptom interview, Saskatoon delirium checklist, delirium rating scale-revised version (DRS-R-98), memorial delirium assessment scale, confusion assessment method, CAM-ICU and clinical assessment of confusion—A and B. CAM has best supported data for its accuracy and ease of use by clinicians. For a comprehensive assessment of delirium, DRS-R-98 has been found to be very useful.

### Confusion Assessment Method (CAM)

It is a 9-item diagnostic instrument and takes only 5 minutes to administer. It captures nine features of delirium which have been grouped into 4 features which includes: features 1 (acute onset and fluctuating course) and 2 (inattention) are essential features, and feature 3 (disorganized thinking) or 4 (altered level of consciousness). It is based on DSM-III R and a diagnosis is made only if the first 2 features and either of the last two features are present. It has been shown to have high concurrent validity when a psychiatrist used it compared to other mental health professionals. However, it has not been found to be useful in the assessment of severity of delirium.

**CAM-ICU** is also a 9-item diagnostic instrument based on DSM-IV and only takes 5 mins to administer. It was mainly developed for patients who are not verbal, can be aroused with voice without any physical stimulation. It has to be administered by trained professionals. It has a high sensitivity and specificity.

**Delirium Rating Scale-revised version (DRS-R-98)** is an oldest, well-known 16 item scale used for assessing the degree of delirium, even in the ICU settings. 3 items are used for helping in the diagnosis and 13 items for assessing the severity on subsequent evaluations. It needs trained professionals to administer the scale. Higher scores suggest higher severity of delirium and the scores are valid for the preceding 24 hrs.

## Dementia Assessments Scales

Currently, there are many scales available to screen, diagnose, assess severity and monitor different domains of cognitive dysfunction. The domains include global impression, specific cognitive domains, activities of daily living, behaviour, quality of life and social interaction. There is also birth of newer scales which captures multiple domains in a single scale called **"multidomain"** scales in Alzheimer's Dementia. Even though it is not the idea of this chapter to review all the scales, we have tried to summarize most of them. For a review of the scales *see* Robert et al 2010.

## i. Screening/shorter Scales

These are brief scales used to screen the cognitive impairment in patients. They usually take 10 to 30 mins to administer and not very comprehensive. Of all the short scales available, mini-mental state examination (MMSE) tops the most for the comprehensive assessments which can be done in a few minutes. The other scales which have almost good psychometric properties like MMSE include 6-CIT, clock drawing and abbreviated mental test score (AMTS) (Sheehan, 2012).

## Mini-Mental State Examination [Folstein, et al. 1975]

The MMSE is a widely used and a comprehensive scale used to assess cognitive impairment in patients. It can be used by physicians and researchers with minimal training. It has 11 items, maximum score of 30 and takes only 10 mins to assess. It assesses 5 broad areas of cognitive functions such as orientation (10 points), registration (3 points), attention and calculation (5 points), recall (3 points), and language (9 points). The cut off score for cognitive impairment is 23 or 24. Some of the limitations of its use are its difficulty in detecting mild to moderate cognitive impairment in people at high educational level or premorbid intelligence ("ceiling" effect) and its inability to detect changes in established advanced dementia, in those with a little formal education and those with severe language problems ("floor" effect) (Franco-Marina, *et al.*, 2010). Another very important drawback of this scale is that it does not capture test frontal/executive or visuospatial (typically right parietal) functions. In order to overcome these properties there have been extended versions of the MMSE Addenbrooke's cognitive examination (ACE), modified mini mental status examination (3MS), cognitive abilities screening instrument (CASI), Cambridge cognitive examination (CAMCOG) and Middlesex elderly assessment memory score (MEAMS).

### Hindi Mental State Examination (HMSE) (Ganguli, et al., 1996)

It is a 22-item screening test intended for illiterate elderly people. It consists of items such as orientation to time and place, three object registration, serial sevens in the form of a story (bus fare), days backwards, three object recall, naming of items, repeat phrase, follow command, three step task, tell me something and copy a diamond within the square. It was developed as part of the Indo-US cross-national dementia epidemiology study but has been shown to be different from MMSE. It has a total score of 30 and a cut-off score of 23 yielded a sensitivity of 94% and specificity 98%.

### Six-Item Cognitive Impairment Test (6CIT) (Brooke and Bullock, 1999)

It is also called Blessed orientation-memory-concentration test, since it was constructed from the 6 items of the Blessed mental status test. It just takes 3 to 4 mins to administer, the scores ranges from 0 to 28 and it was primarily designed to be used in primary care settings. It has one memory, two calculations and three orientations items and a cut-off of 7/8 showing good screening sensitivity and specificity.

### Clock Drawing Test (CDT)

It screens for frontal/executive, visuospatial and constructional praxis impairment. The test involves a patient to draw a clock face with numbers and hands (indicating a dictated time usually 10 past 11). There are many scoring methods; a simple one uses one mark each for a correctly drawn circle; appropriately spaced numbers; and hands that show the right time summating to a maximum score of 3. The advantage of this test is not only the timing but also freedom from any biases from culture or language or intellectual capacity.

### Abbreviated Mental Test Score (AMTS)

It is a 10-item scale which assesses the orientation, registration, recall and concentration. A cut-off less than 6 suggests significant cognitive deficits. It takes only 3 to 4 mins to administer and has been used both in primary and secondary settings in elderly patients.

### ii. Longer Scales

### Alzheimer's Disease Assessment Scale—Cognitive Section (Rosen, et al. 1984)

It is a detailed cognitive and non-cognitive AD-specific scale and has to be used by trained professionals. There are 11 subtests which assess memory, praxis, and language (cognitive) and 10 items which evaluate mood and behavioural changes (non-cognitive). Since this scale also have ceiling, floor effects and lacks certain other important tests; a newly added test Neuropsychological Test Battery (NTB) fills the limitations.

### The Cambridge Assessment of Memory and Cognition (Roth, et al. 1986)

It is the cognitive section of the comprehensive assessment scale called CAMDEX. It assesses orientation, language, memory, attention, praxis, calculation, abstract thinking and perception. It takes 25–40 min and has a cut-offs of 79/80 for dementia.

*Kolkata Cognitive Screening Battery (Das, et al. 2006)*

It is a screening test battery which consists of category-based verbal fluency tests (fruits and animals), a 15-item version of the object naming test, mental state examination, calculation tests, visuo-constructional ability which included drawing the circle, diamond, overlapping rectangles, box and a set of memory tests which consisted of immediate memory, delayed and recognition of a 10-item word list. It has been used and validated by Ganguli, et al. in a rural population and by Das et al in urban population.

*PGI Battery of Brain Dysfunction (Pershad and Verma, 1990)*

It is standardized battery for screening cognitive dysfunction and also used for other neuropsychological assessment. It assesses cognitive functions in the domains of intelligence, memory and perceptuo-motor functions. It consists of the following subtests: Verbal Adult Intelligence Scale, Revised Bhatia's Short Battery of Performance Tests of Intelligence, PGI Memory Scale, Nahor and Benson Test: a measure of perceptuo-motor functions and Bender Visuo-Motor Gestalt Test: A measure of perceptuo-motor functions.

*PGI Memory Test*

It is a subtest of the PGI Battery of Brain Dysfunction and a standardized test to measure verbal and nonverbal memory. It has ten subtests which use verbal and nonverbal material and measures remote memory, recent memory, mental balance, attention and concentration (digit span), delayed recall, immediate recall, verbal retention for similar pairs, verbal retention for dissimilar pairs, visual retention, and recognition. The total scores of 10 subtests will be used to calculate percentile ratio as more than 40 and less than or equal to 40. It has norms for general population and has been extensively used in Indian studies.

*NIMHANS Neuropsychological Battery for Elderly (NNBE) (Tripathi, 2012)*

Initially a general neuropsychological battery called NIMHANS Neuropsychological Battery (NNB) was developed in NIMHANS by Rao SL, Subbakrishnan DK, Gopulkumar K (2004). It captured some of the important cognitive functions such as tests of speed, attention, Memory, Executive Function and Comprehension. Most of the tests were taken from other standardized battery of tests, such as the Luria-Nebraska Neuropsychological battery.

Recently, Tripathi developed the NIMHANS Neuropsychological Battery for Elderly (NNBE) which is a brief (60 mins), comprehensive and standardized neuropsychological battery for older Indian adults. It assesses Episodic memory (word list), immediate, delayed recall and memory of logical passage (story recall test), attention (span task and picture cancellation task), visuospatial constructional ability (stick construction test), executive functions (digit span, Corsi block-tapping test, fluency and Go/No-Go task and Tower of Hanoi), language (picture naming test and semantic verbal fluency test), parietal focal signs (agnosia/apraxia/body schema disturbances /left right disorientation/acalcuila).

### iii. Activities Of Daily Living (ADL) Scales

There are around 17 questionnaires available to assess the functional ability of dementia patients. It covers basic ADL such as feeding, dressing, walking to complex activities such as using telephone, cooking, shopping and transportation (instrumental ADL). The most commonly scale used is Katz Index of ADL which covers 6 basic ADL such as feeding, bathing, dressing, toileting, transfer and continence. A review of all the scales has opined that disability assessment for dementia (DAD) (gelinas, et al. 1999) and the Bristol activities of daily living Scale (Bucks, et al. 1996) had better ratings than the rest.

#### Indian Disability Evaluation Assessment Scale (IDEAS)

IDEAS is a general disability scale for psychiatric patients and not specific for elderly with cognitive impairment. It was developed by the rehabilitation committee of the Indian Psychiatric society. It assesses the individual under four domains: self-care, interpersonal activities (social relationships), communication and understanding, and occupation, including performance at employment/housework/education. Each item is scored between 0 and 4, i.e. from no to profound disability.

Adding the scores on the four items gives the 'total disability score'.

## iv. Behaviour

Recently many scales are available to assess the behavioural problems in patients with dementia. Some of the important scales which are commonly used include BEHAVE-AD, Neuropsychiatric Inventory (NPI) and Cohen-Mansfield Agitation Inventory. BEHAVE-AD (Reisberg, et al. 1987) is a clinician administered scale based on observation and self-report. It takes 20 mins to administer the scale and covers important symptoms such as, activity disturbances, aggressiveness, affective disorders, hallucinations, paranoid and delusional ideation, diurnal rhythm disturbances, and anxieties, and phobias. NPI (Cummings, et al. 1994) is an informant-based scale to assess wide range of behavioural disturbances such as irritability, apathy, disinhibition, delusions, agitation and depression. It overcame some of the items missed in BEHAVE-AD.

## v. Quality Of Life Scales

The quality of life scales are based on the Lawton's model of QoL in dementia and reports that the QoL is based on the dynamic interaction between four patient-relevant dimensions: Psychological well-being, perceived quality of life, behaviour competence, and environment. There are many dementia specific scales available which include the quality of life—Alzheimer's disease (QoL-AD), DEMQOL, Alzheimer Disease related quality of life (ADRQL), the dementia quality of life instrument (DQoL) and the quality of life in late-stage dementia scale (QUALID).

Quality of life—Alzheimer's disease (QoL—AD) (Logsdon, et al. 1999) is a 13-item well-validated scale which can be used in all the severity of dementia patients. It takes just 15 mins to administer and can be completed by the patient or the care-giver.

DEMQOL (Smith, et al. 2007) is a 31-item scale which assesses the health-related quality of life and which has been well validated with other scales.

## 2. DEPRESSION RATING SCALES

There are numerous scales, specific and non-specific scales, used to assess depression in the elderly. There are barriers in using these scales in the elderly, they include over representation of somatic symptoms, cognitive impairment, visual and hearing impairment and comorbid medical complications. Some of the non-specific scales used are the Hamilton depression rating scale [Hamilton,1960] , Montgomery Asberg depression rating scale (MADRS) [Montgomery and Asberg, 1979] and the hospital anxiety and depression scale [Zigmond and Snaith, 1983]. The specific scales such as the geriatric depression scale (GDS) [Yesavage*et al.* 1983], the Cornell scale for depression in dementia (CSDD) [Alexopoulos, et al. 1988a], brief assessment schedule depression cards (BASDEC), and the geriatric mental state schedule (GMSS). The gold standard scales to assess depression in the elderly is the Geriatric depression scale (GDS) and specifically in dementia is Cornell scale for depression in dementia (CSDD).

**Geriatric depression scale (GDS-15)** is a short form, self-rated, 15-item scale and takes only 5 to 10 mins to administer. It has been validated mainly patients with mild dementia and not for those with moderate to severe. It is available in many languages and can be used by telephonic conversation also.

**Cornell scale for depression in dementia (CSDD)** is a 19-item scale which can be administered in the patient and the caregiver. It has been validated in elderly with and without dementia.

### 3. CARER BURDEN SCALE

Caregiver's burden is a very important aspect to be addressed in elderly patients with cognitive deficits. Early recognition and help offered to them may prevent verbal and physical abuse, neglect of the elderly, burnout in the carer and interpersonal problems. General Health Questionnaire and Zarit Burden Interview [Zarit, et al. 1980] have been used in caregivers to assess their distress.

The **Zarit burden interview** is a 22-item, self-report inventory which assess the subjective burden among caregivers of adults with dementia. Each item has a likert type of scoring from never to nearly always present. The total scores ranges from 0 (low burden) to 88 (high burden).

## LABORATORY INVESTIGATIONS AND NEUROIMAGING

Elderly patients are very vulnerable to cognitive dysfunction due to subtle changes in metabolic parameters. It is important to assess for the etiology of cognitive dysfunctions in them. Sometimes all the parameters may be normal, then specific battery of specialized tests may be required whenever there is some suspicion of some underlying pathology. The investigations should be based on clues obtained from the detailed history and physical examination. In a low income country like India, where most of the elderly are having less financial resources and no public insurances; investigations should be judiciously used. The investigations are summarized in Tables 11.1–11.3 as (1) routine/essential investigations (2) specialized investigations and (3) imaging.

| Table 11.1: Routine investigations | |
|---|---|
| *Test* | *Indication/usefulness* |
| Complete blood count | • To look for general health conditions<br>• Iron deficiency, anemia and Infections |
| Erythrocyte sedimentation rate | • For signs of inflammation in the body |
| ALT or AST/GGT | • Liver status, alcohol induced liver dysfunction |
| Blood urea and serum creatinine | • Kidney function test |
| Electrolytes | • Deficiencies and kidney functions |
| Fasting and postprandial | • Level of sugar in the blood. |
| Glycated hemo-globin (HbA1C) | • To monitor for blood sugar control and to identify for microvascular disease<br>• People with diabetes may require once in 3 months |

Contd.

| Table 11.1: Routine investigations (Contd.) | |
|---|---|
| *Test* | *Indication/usefulness* |
| Serum albumin | • To help determine protein and immune status. |
| Lipid profile | • To determine risk level for CVD |
| TSH | • To check for the activity of thyroid |
| Uric acid | • To diagnose and monitor patients with gout<br>• monitor patients undergoing chemotherapy or radiation treatment<br>• To diagnose kidney disorders and monitor its function post-injury<br>• Determine the cause of kidney stones |
| $FT_3$ and $FT_4$ | • If TSH shows any abnormalities, to further assess hypothyroidism or hyperthyroidism or sub-clinical hypothyroidism |
| Prostate-specific antigen (PSA) in men | • To rule out prostatitis or prostate cancer |
| Phosphorus | • To rule out parathyroid disease |
| Urinalysis | • Vital test for infections, microalbuminuria, specific gravity and ketone bodies |
| VDRL and HIV | • To rule out sexually transmitted diseases<br>• To find the etiology in case of syphilitic encephalitis or HIV dementia |
| Serum ammonia | • To rule out liver abnormalities in delirium or drug induced hyperammonemia (Valproate) |
| Mammography and pap smear in women | • To rule out breast cancer or cervical cancers in women |
| Pulse oximetry or arterial blood gases | • Hypoxemia |

| Table 11.2: Specialized investigations | |
|---|---|
| *Test* | *Indication/usefulness* |
| Vitamin B$_{12}$, folate and homocysteine | • Treatable causes of dementia and neuropsychiatric disorders<br>• In vegetarians with indications of achlorhydria and gastrointestinal problems<br>• Hyperhomocysteinemia is associated with increased risk of occlusive vascular disease, thrombosis, stroke and cognitive dysfunction |
| HIV | • To rule out HIV-related cognitive disorder/dementia |
| Urine drug screen | • To detect for drugs of abuse causing delirium or other cognitive dysfunction (amnestic disorders, e.g. Wernicke's Encephalopathy) |
| Toxicology screen | • For detecting drugs or heavy metals leading to delirium or dementia |
| 24 hr cortisol | • To rule out Cushing's disease |
| Porphobilinogen and ALA in 24 hr urine | • To rule out acute intermittent porphyria |
| Cortrosyn stimulating test | • To rule out Addison's disease |
| Ceruloplasmin | • To rule out Wilson's diseases |
| Anti-nuclear antibodies | • To diagnose autoimmune diseases |
| Cerebrospinal fluid (CSF) | • To study the cell cytology to detect infections (e.g. tuberculosis) or inflammation |
| Electroen-cephalogram (EEG) | • Distinguish dementia from delirium based on the EEG waves and to look for unusual brain activity found in Creutzfeldt-Jakob disease, a rare cause of dementia |

Contd.

| **Table 11.2:** Specialized investigations (Contd.) | |
|---|---|
| *Test* | *Indication/usefulness* |
| Genetic Testing *APOE* | • Mutations on chromosome 1, 14 and 21 linked to rare forms of early-onset familial Alzheimer's disease<br>• *APOEε4* allele associated with increased risk for Alzheimer's disease<br>• Ethical issues in the use of these tests in asymptomatic individuals. |
| Brain biopsy | • If a treatable cause of dementia is suspected (to consider a biopsy).<br>• After death, to confirm the diagnosis of the etiology of dementia for the families wanting to know the genetic etiology. |

| **Table 11.3:** Imaging | |
|---|---|
| *Test* | *Indication/usefulness* |
| Plain Film radiographs | • To detect lung pathology, bone fractures |
| ECG | • To detect for any cardiovascular disorders and monitor for conduction disorders and QTc interval due to psychiatric medications |
| Ultra sound abdomen | • To rule out any tumours of the abdomen |
| Computed Tomography (CT) | • Useful in detecting bone abnormalities, areas of hemorrhage, Brain atrophy, ventricular enlargement, and mass effect due to lesions |
| Magnetic Resonance Imaging (MRI) | • High resolution images and good details of posterior fossa<br>• Brain tumours, strokes, normal-pressure hydrocephalus, midbrain hemorrhage (Wernicke's encephalopathy) |

Contd.

| Table 11.3: Imaging (Contd.) | |
|---|---|
| *Test* | *Indication/Usefulness* |
| | or other conditions that could cause dementia symptoms. |
| Diffusion weighted Imaging (DWI) | • To differentiate acute vs chronic lesions<br>• In the brain which may not be possible with CT or MRI |
| Single photon emission CT (SPECT) and PET scan | • To identify several forms of dementia, including vascular dementia and frontotemporal dementia. |

## Sample Images

Image 1.  CT scan showing right hemispheric bleeds
Image 2.  MRI showing acute large left MAC infarct with hemorrhagic transformation

## PSYCHOSOCIAL ISSUES

### Socio-demographic Profile

India has the second largest aged population in the world next to China. The population of the elderly (>60 yrs) in India has been estimated to be 102 million in 2011 and it has been projected to double by 2050. Most of the elderly population are males (51.8%) but most of the women are widowed (55%) due to increased life expectancy of women. It has been estimated that most of them in this category reside in the rural area (75%) and have high old age dependency ratio (12.5%) compared to urban. Most of the dependent elderly are supported by their children and grandchildren. The elderly are more dependent on the male children but the trend is currently changing to female children.

### Social Issues

India was synonymous with joint family; elders had the authority and were the decision makers. Currently, it is slowly changing to the point of disappearing and there are only a few joint families in the urban areas (< 5%). Some of the reasons for this include rapid industrialization, urbanization, rapid growth of population, improvement in transport and communication, influence of other cultures and decline in agriculture. The younger generations are well educated, economically independent and have taken over the authority and decision-making power of the elderly. Even though most of the younger generation feels that they are a burden to them; a few of them report that having an elderly person at home is very helpful in taking decisions, help during the times of sickness, advice in family matters, education and all-round development of the family. Some of them even dump their parents in old age homes and don't care for them.

### Economic Issues

Physiological changes in them reduces their capacity to work and earn. There is a general opinion that elderly are not employed and dependent on their children in India. In fact it is not true, it is reported that 40% of the elderly (both genders) are working and 61% of the elderly male are more economically active. But the irony is that 90% of them who work are dependent on unorganized sector. Due to this they retire without any pension, financial resources, medical benefits or other concessions. This makes them more vulnerable and dependent on others.

### Health Problems

Ageing makes them more vulnerable to medical illnesses, disability and psychiatric/psychological problems. Cardiac disorders, high blood pressure, arthritis, rheumatism and urinary problems are the most prevalent chronic diseases in them. Some of the disabilities faced by them include problems in mobility, blindness (partial or complete), deafness (partial or complete), breathlessness, memory disturbances and indigestion.

### Psychological Aspects

The concept of self changes as a person starts ageing. They have to accept that their body is not as energetic as before, financial resources are low, and dependence on spouse or children is a must, no freedom of decision making, loss of loved ones, cognitive slowing and physiological changes of the body. These can cause significant negative image and poor coping or adjustment. Indian researchers have found a few determinants of successful ageing, they include self-acceptance of ageing changes, self-perception of health, perceived functional ability, perception of social support, inter-generational amity, belief in karma and afterlife, flexibility, range of interests, activity level, marital satisfaction, religiosity, certain value orientations and economic well-being. (Ramamurti and Jamuna, 1992, Niharika, 2004, Siva Raju, 2006).

### Elderly Female

Globally, women live longer than males and become more dependent on others, become widowed, have poor financial resources and become caretakers of their husband. These aspects can lead to physical illness and mental stress.

### Abuse

Elderly persons are more prone to physical and verbal abuse than others. Those who are at high risk include females (advanced age), role-less, functionally impaired, lonely and living at home (with their adult child, spouse or other relatives). The most common type of abuse includes psychological abuse in terms of verbal assaults, threats and fear of isolation, physical violence, neglect and financial exploitation. They are also more vulnerable for crime and it ranges from simple hurt, robbery, murder to severe crimes such as sexual assaults. Most of the crimes have occurred in the elderly females, indoors, during daytime and 25% of the perpetrators are their own family members.

### Conclusion

It is important to know that India is growing with the elderly population and has been termed the "Ageing" country. With all the issues discussed above, are we prepared to take care of the problems faced by them? The geriatric medicine is still in the nascent stages of development. We need to have more services and research in this area to help the elderly. Old age is their second childhood; we need to give back what they gave the youngsters in their childhood.

**ORGANIC CONDITIONS**

## DELIRIUM

It is a neuropsychiatric syndrome with an acute onset with a transient, fluctuating course which is usually reversible. It has been retained in the DSM-V, in the neurocognitive disorders. It is characterized by disturbances in consciousness, orientation, memory, perception, thought and behaviour. The core symptoms of delirium are attention deficits, motor activity changes and disturbances of sleep-wake cycle. The other features such as psychotic symptoms, mood symptoms, memory impairment and language disturbances are variable in presentation (*see* Table 11.4 for differences between delirium and dementia). It is one of the commonest presentations in the elderly psychiatric referrals. In India, the prevalence of delirium in the elderly (> 65 yrs) in India has ranged from 3 to 27%. There are three types of delirium which include hypoactive, hyperactive and mixed. A persistent variety has also been described where patients from delirium do not recover and has been associated with poor outcome. Some of the risk factors for its development include pre-existing cognitive deficits, postoperative period, hip fractures, longer duration of surgery, neurological illnesses, urinary tract infections, visual impairment, hearing impairment, current pneumonia, leucocytosis, raised blood ammonia, hyponatremia and hypo/hyperkalaemia. Even though the exact etiology is not clear, various hypotheses have been presented. They include neurotransmitter hypothesis, cholinergic hypothesis, dopamine excess hypothesis, reduction of plasma activity of cholinesterases and inflammation or acute stress response (increased cytokines due to surgery, trauma or infection and high levels of cortisol). Most authors concur that a single molecule or factor cannot explain the etiology of delirium and a simple heuristic approach is required. Delirium has been associated with poor prognosis in terms of increased hospital stay, cognitive decline, functional decline, institutionalization, prolonged use of mechanical ventilation (ICU) and mortality.

The management involves investigations and treatment. Delirium is a medical emergency and better managed in a medical ward or in an ICU setting depending on the severity. A brief history into the onset of symptoms and probable etiology has to be elicited (infections, medication, substance use, trauma, worsening of medical conditions, physiological/ metabolic abnormalities and at times neoplasms/secondaries in the brain). Lab investigations such as complete blood count (including ESR), electrolytes, urine analysis, kidney and liver function test, blood sugars, thyroid function test, serum ammonia ( suspected hepatic encephalopathy or drug induced hyperammonemia), VDRL and HIV (to rule out syphilis or AIDS) and CT or MRI may be required. For a detailed lab investigation see Tables in Section Lab investigations. Treatment involves pharmacological and non-pharmacological interventions. Non-pharmacological treatment involves looking into etiology of the delirium, supportive care, education of the family members, environmental manipulation, preventing complications and treating behavioural problems. Before starting any treatment involving the family members in treatment decisions are very important. Their role in calming the patient, orienting them, supporting and protecting them during procedures can be very soothing for the patient. Supportive care involves continued care from the nursing staff in monitoring vital signs, good nutrition, adequate fluid balance, preventing falls or aspiration, cleanliness and good body hygiene and maintaining good sleep pattern. Physical restrain is rarely used and only when the patients are very agitated and to be strictly avoided routinely. Environmental manipulation involves providing a comfortable place and a well lit room for the patient. The room should have a large clock with a calendar to re-orient the patient frequently and reducing sensory deprivation. It is very important to avoid frequent change of nursing personnel, sensory overload or keep the patient in open spaces. Pharmacological treatment is mainly intended for behavioural management such as agitation or not co-operating for medical procedures. Recent guidelines recommend use of haloperidol or olanzapine in low doses and based on the improvement to gradually titrate the doses. Parental injections can be used in violent or agitated patients.

In conclusion, delirium is a medical emergency and needs to be addressed. Brief history looking into the etiology and treatment of the cause can relieve the symptoms faster. Non-pharmacological treatments are as important as that of pharmacological treatment which are mainly used for behavioural problems.

## MILD COGNITIVE IMPAIRMENT (MCI)

In clinical conditions many a times we face situations where the patients may have subtle cognitive problems such as forgetting, not able to find objects or difficulty in remembering the names. They or their family members may present to doctors with the anxiety that they may have dementia. It is important to note that not all patients with the above symptoms have dementia but may fall into a category called mild cognitive impairment (MCI). Petersen (2004) defined MCI as an *objective impairment on neuropsychological tests, with maintenance of intact global cognitive functioning and activities of daily living*. Earlier it was called by different names such as benign senescent forgetfulness, aging-associated cognitive, decline, age-associated memory impairment, late-life forgetfulness and cognitive impairment, no dementia but currently the term MCI is used commonly.

There are a lot of controversies in the criteria for MCI. In 1999, Peterson et al proposed a diagnostic criterion which included subjective memory complaint, retained independence in activities of daily living, abnormal memory for age, typically 1.5 SD below peers, and normal general cognitive function and the criteria for dementia must not be met. However, it was later modified and the focus shifted from specific memory complaint to general cognitive deficit. Based on these modifications, they classified MCI into amnestic mild cognitive impairment (aMCI) (with single and multiple domain variants) and non-amnestic MCI (naMCI) (with single and multiple domain variants). However, the concept is still evolving.

The estimation of prevalence of MCI has faced huge problems since there are no consensuses on the definition. Generally the age associated memory impairment has ranged from 17 to 36%, while the age associated cognitive decline has been found to be 26%. In India, Das et al (2007) found a prevalence of 14.89% in 960 subjects aged over 50 yrs in Kolkata.

Multiple risk factors have been identified which have been associated with MCI. Some of the poor risk factor include presence of APOE-4, African American ethnicity, early cognitive deficits, cortical atrophy, hypertension, diabetes mellitus, cardiac diseases (coronary heart disease, congestive cardiac failure and atrial fibrillation), poor pulmonary function (low $FEV_1/$ height$^2$ ratio at baseline), anticholinergic drug use and depression. However, moderate exercise and higher educational levels have been found to have lesser risk on MCI.

Individuals diagnosed to have MCI may remain stable or may show improvement on cognitive tests on follow-up or may progress to dementia. There has been wide variation in the conversions and is probably due to differences in the criteria used for defining MCI. Most studies have reported a range of 6.5 to 12% annual conversion to dementia and differential rates of 6.5% for AD and 1.6% for VD. Later studies reported that aMCI had 48.7% and naMCI had 26.8% conversion rates in a cohort of 581 subjects. This emphasized that compared to subjects with aMCI; naMCI may actually progress to AD which has changed the conventional thinking of aMCI. Also, measures of delayed recall have been found to be best neuropsychological predictors of conversion of MCI to dementia. These need to be considered along with strict criteria for the definition of MCI and dementia.

Neuroimaging studies have many attempts to study the early changes in the brain regions to predict MCI using magnetic resonance imaging (MRI), magnetic resonance spectroscopy (MRS), electroencephalogram (EEG) and positron emission tomography (PET). Most studies confirmed pathological changes in the hippocampal volume and reported that the conversion rate to dementia was 9%. It has also been noted that size of hippocampus was inversely proportional to the dementia risk. Further studies found that the atrophy of the CA1 region within the hippocampus compared to other areas was associated with higher risk of conversion. Some authors have also found significant difference in the mediodorsal aspect of the entorhinal cortex and the mid-parietal portion of the parahippocampal gyrus in MCI converters compared to non-converters. Using EEG technique, Moretti et al found that increased theta/gamma wave ratio and increased alpha3/alpha2 ratio were statistically elevated in those individuals with MCI who converted to AD. Using PET, it is possible to demonstrate the extent of b-amyloid deposition in the brain but the research is still in the infancy and it is not currently recommended.

Cognitive assessments used for screening MCI include Addenbrooke's Cognitive Examination Revised edition (ACE-R), DemTect and Montreal Cognitive Assessment (MoCA). ACE-R has been able to show the difference in tests of memory, verbal fluency and language in subjects with MCI compared to Controls. DemTect is a simple and objective test which contains five tasks to assess the verbal memory, verbal fluency, intellectual flexibility and attention. The total scores ranges from 0 to 18 and a score of 8 or less for dementia, 9–12 for MCI and 13 and above for normal performance. MoCA is a simple, 30-point screening test which assesses the short-term memory, visuospatial abilities, executive functions, language, attention, orientation and working memory. Free and Cued Selective Recall Reminding Test and tests of executive function are likely to help in detecting MCI. However, MMSE has not been found to be a good tool to help in the screening of MCI.

Currently there are no effective pharmacological agents for the treatment of MCI. In fact it is recommended not to use acetylcholinesterase inhibitors in MCI. Many non-pharmacological methods have been suggested such as improved diet, blood pressure lowering medication in patients with hypertension (without cerebrovascular disease) and resistance training. However, most guidelines suggest regular follow-up in this group, so that early treatment can be instituted to prevent further progression.

## DEMENTIA

Dementia is not specific disorder or a normal progression of ageing but it is a clinical syndrome characterized by progressive deterioration of cognitive functioning such as memory, thinking, orientation, comprehension, calculation, learning capacity, language, and judgement and it impairs the normal functioning and quality of life. It can be classified based on the clinical presentation, etiology or neuropathology findings.

The prevalence of dementia worldwide is 35.6 million (2010) and is projected to increase to 115.4 million in 2050. In India, the prevalence of dementia in 2010 was 3.7 million (> 60 yrs) and 2.1 million of them are women and the rest were men. Of all the Indian states, Trivandrum (Kerala) and Thirupur (Tamil Nadu) had highest rates compared to Ballabgarh and Vellore which had the lowest rates of dementia.

It can be grouped grossly into four types which include (1) Alzheimer's dementia (AD)(early and late onset); (2) the Parkinson's group (Lewy body disease, dementia of Parkinson's and Alzheimer's dementia with Parkinson's); (3) the Frontotemporal group (behavioural variant of FTD (bvFTD), semantic dementia (SD) and progressive non-fluent aphasia (PNFA) and Pick's disease) and (4) the vascular group (large and small vessel disease).

The etiology of the dementia includes neurodegenerative, vascular, intracranial space occupying lesions, metabolic, endocrine, traumatic brain injury, epilepsy, infections, toxic, hypoxia, vitamin deficiency and rare causes.

## Dementia Due to Alzheimer's Disease (AD)

Dementia due to Alzheimer's disease (AD) is the commonest type of dementia and ranges from 50 to 70% compared to other types. The second most common is vascular dementia which is a heterogeneous group. There are two types of AD, which includes (1) Early-onset familial—they develop symptoms before the age of 65 years and (2) Late-onset—develop symptoms after the age of 65 years.

## Clinical Features in AD

**Memory disturbances**: It occurs in early stages and usually occurs for the recent events; however, the remote and working memories are spared. In early stages, the patient may be able to repeat the three items suggesting intact working memory but may not be able to recall the three items after 5 minutes while they are distracted. They also have difficulties in learning new memories and storage compared to other types of dementias with memory difficulties. Thus, suggesting that the primary problems with the memory in AD is storing and encoding rather than retrieval problems. Semantic memory, which is the understanding and knowledge about the words, facts and concept are initially preserved but as the disease progresses, it worsens. Visuospatial dysfunctions present as disorientation in strange places and getting lost in familiar places.

**Aphasias:** In the early stages of AD, they may have subtle difficulties in language which may be easier for the family members to identify. They also have word finding difficulty, incomplete sentences, grammatical errors and poor use of tenses in the early stages. In the later aspect of the disease, they have receptive difficulties, perseverations, echolalia and decreased fluency. They may try to compensate by different strategies.

**Apraxia:** In the early stages they may have ideomotor apraxia and they have difficulties in complex motor tasks without a primary motor difficulty. They have difficulties such as enacting a command in a detailed and goal directed acts and this manifests as poor self-care, poor ADL and can harm themselves.

**Agnosia:** They have difficulty in recognise one's own face (autoprosopagnosia) which is due to difficulty in correctly interpreting sensory input.

**Executive dysfunction:** Executive functioning is the primary frontal lobe function. The ability to plan, organize and sustain attention is affected early in AD.

**Activities of Daily Living (ADL):** There are two types: (1) Basic (self-care) and (2) Instrumental. Dysfunction of the ADL is associated with the cognitive dysfunction and is a criterion for diagnosis of AD in DSM-IV. The instrumental ADL is actually affected early than the Basic ADL. Initially, they have predominantly difficulties in finding personal belongings, later it progresses to difficulties only in demanding circumstances and in terminal stages they may bed bound.

**Behavioural and Psychological Symptoms of Dementia (BPSD):** The behavioural and psychological symptoms can be grouped into three groups: **(1) Psychotic (2) Mood (3) Activity related. Psychotic symptoms** usually occur in one-third of AD patients but it is not clear whether it is in the early or late phase. Psychotic symptoms are associated with depression and aggression. Some of the common psychotic symptoms include hallucinations, delusions and misidentification syndrome. Of all the symptoms delusions are the common psychotic symptoms and usually the theme is of theft or stealing. They have a complex explanation for how the theft occurred and are secondary to the memory disturbances (not true delusions). The common types of hallucinations include visual but other types are also present. It involves visualizing small animals or people; they have insight about it and are usually silent and fearless. In the misidentification syndrome, the AD patients are able to identify the face (different from prosopagnosia) and believe that an imposter has replaced them. **Mood symptoms** are also common in AD. The prevalence of anxiety (>50%) and depression (10–25%) are common compared to mania (<5%). Depressive symptoms are more commonly seen than major depression. They have found that in patients with AD having depression, there is a loss of neurons in locus coeruleusand probably the dorsal raphe nucleus suggesting loss of serotonergic and noradrenergic functions. The frequency of disturbances in **activity** is also common in AD. They include apathy, agitation, wandering, aggression and circadian rhythm disturbances.

## Diagnosis

A possible diagnosis of AD is mainly based on clinical criteria and a probable diagnosis is based only on biomarkers and postmortem study of the brain of AD. Hence, the clinical history and information given by the relatives is very vital in the diagnosis of dementia. The most common diagnostic criteria used is diagnostic and statistical manual of mental disorders, 4th edition (DSM-IV). However, with the introduction of DSM-V in 2014, there are a few updates in the classification. They include change in the terminology of dementia to "major neurocognitive disorder (NCD)", and a less severe level of cognitive impairment, termed "mild NCD". Also, the National Institute on Aging and Alzheimer's Association has suggested new diagnostic guidelines. They define three stages of AD which include (1) Preclinical phase: Neuropathologic changes occur, no overt (or only subtle) symptoms (2) Phase of mild cognitive impairment: Symptoms become apparent; ADL are preserved; the patient does not have dementia (3) Dementia phase: ADL are impaired.

Once a diagnosis of dementia is made; it is important to identify for any treatable causes of dementia. Appropriate lab investigations and imaging has to be done to exclude the causes. It is also important to assess the cognitive functions using screening and rating scales. An attempt should be made to assess the daily functioning of the patient. Then determine the presence and degree of behavioural symptoms in them. It is also very important to identify for the primary caregiver's knowledge and burden, if any. The role of family and other support systems are very important and have to be assessed if it is adequate.

## Pharmacotherapy

The Food and Drug Administration (FDA) has approved a few medications for AD. It is important to know that the medications may improve symptoms or delay decline but they do not improve the underlying neurodegenerative process. This has to be communicated to the patients and family members. The medications include Cholinesterase Inhibitors (Donepezil, Galantamine and Rivastigmine) which are indicated for mild-to-moderate AD; Rivastigmine transdermal patch has been specifically indicated for severe AD and NMDA receptor antagonist (Memantine) which is indicated for moderate-to-severe AD.

## Medical Foods

Now, medical foods are available for the management of AD and/or cognitive impairment. It is important to note that there are no data supporting the effectiveness of medical foods since they have not undergone a rigorous scientific scrutiny as approved drugs and there are no premarketing review process available. Some of the formulations available currently include **Caprylidene** (a proprietary formulation of medium-chain triglycerides, intended for dietary management of mild to moderate AD), **Cerefolin NAC** (combination of folic acid, vitamin $B_{12}$, and N-acetylcysteine, intended for dietary management of mild cognitive impairment), **Vayacog** (a combination of phosphatidylserine, docosahexaenoic acid, and eicosapentaenoic acid, intended for dietary management of lipid imbalances associated with early memory impairment) and **Souvenaid** (combination of omega-3 fatty acids, uridine, choline, vitamins C, E, $B_6$, and $B_{12}$, selenium, and folic acid , is indicated for mild AD and intended for dietary means of supporting synaptic integrity).

### Non-Pharmacological Therapy

There are lots of therapies available for people with dementia. They can be classified into standard, alternative and brief psychotherapies. The **standard therapies** include behavioural therapy, cognitive stimulation, ADL training, reality orientation, validation therapy and reminiscence therapy. The **alternative therapies include** art therapy, music therapy, pet therapy, recreation therapy, acupuncture, transcranial magnetic stimulation, muscle relaxation, physical exercise, massage and touch, complementary therapy, aromatherapy, bright-light therapy and multisensory approaches. The **brief psychotherapies include** cognitive behavioural therapy, interpersonal therapy.

It is also important to address the problems of the care-givers. Some of the interventions include caregiver education, caregiver support, case management, and respite care.

### Conclusion

There are lots of advances occurring in the field of dementia. Researchers are working on the early intervention, neuroimaging, pharmacological treatments, guidelines and non-invasive interventions. In the coming decades, we hope to understand the etiology of dementia and develop newer treatment modalities.

## PSYCHIATRIC DISORDERS IN ELDERLY

### DEPRESSION IN THE ELDERLY

Depression was the leading cause of WHO Global Burden of Diseases in 2000–2002 and it is projected to become the leading disorder of the disability adjusted life years in 2030. Globally, the prevalence of depression in the elderly ranged from 10 to 20% (WHO). In India, very few studies have been done on large population. In the community studies the prevalence has ranged from 13 to 25% and in PHC it has ranged from 10 to 25%. A higher prevalence of geriatric depression (21.9 %) was found in India in a meta-analysis of 74 studies worldwide.

Elderly patients presented with more of hypochondriacal complaints, medically unexplained symptoms, agitation and depressive delusions compared to younger depressives. The different types of depression seen in elderly include major depression (single or recurrent), psychotic depression, bipolar depression, dysthymia, brief or subsyndromal depression, bereavement, adjustment disorder, depression in patients with dementia, pseudodementia, depression-executive dysfunction syndrome (DED), depression associated with medical disorders and subcortical ischemic depression (SID) (major depression with magnetic resonance imaging (MRI) evidence of subcortical lesions) (see Table 11.5 for differences between pseudodementia and dementia).

Suicide is twice as common in elderly compared to general population. Some of the factors associated with high risk of suicide include high severity of depression, psychotic depression, alcoholism, recent bereavement, abuse of sedatives, and recent development of disability are the most important risk factors in depressed elderly.

Longitudinal studies have reported that 7 to 30% of the elderly have chronic major depression. Naturalistic treatment studies report 13 to 19 % of the elderly relapse or have a recurrence at one year but if they are on controlled antidepressant treatment, then their relapse rate is 15%.

The evaluation of depression in the elderly should focus on organic causes and include evaluation of psychopathology, medical history, medication history, neurological status, functional impairment and psychosocial stressors. A complete blood count, TSH, AST/ALT, vitamin $B_{12}$ and serum electrolytes are some of the important lab tests needed in the elderly with depression. Neuroimaging may be considered in first onset of depression in the elderly (for a detailed evaluation of lab investigation see the topic on lab investigation).

SSRI's have become the first line of treatment for mild to moderate depression in the elderly. It has been effective even in the elderly with stroke, vascular diseases and Alzheimer's dementia. It does not have anticholinergic, orthostatic, cardiac side-effects, oversedation which is often associated with tricyclic antidepressants (TCAs) and are also safe in overdoses. They have different types of side-effects such as activation, sleep disturbances, gastritis, headache or worsening of migraine, hyponatremia, weight loss and GI side-effects. The next line of medication if the SSRI's are not effective or not tolerated are venlafaxine or duloxetine. However, it is important to remember that those on higher doses of venlafaxine can have increased heart rate and blood pressure and duloxetine can cause urinary retention which can be bothersome side effects. However, in elderly who are not improving with the above treatment and have major depression, TCA's may be tried with caution. However, the elderly need to be able to tolerate the side effects such as anticholinergic and sedation. If the elderly are not improving with TCA's, then newer antidepressants such as trazodone, bupropion can be considered and they do not have anticholinergic side effects. If none of the above medications are effective, then modified electroconvulsive therapy can be considered and they are especially useful in agitated depression. Certain precautions have to be taken, such as benzodiazepine should be avoided and reserpine and anticholinesterase should be withdrawn.

*Note of caution:* Some of the elderly patients who may be on anti-diuretics for hypertension and for other reasons, SSRIs can contribute to sodium loss and its consequences.

Among psychotherapies, cognitive behavioural therapy, interpersonal therapy and problem-solving therapy have been found to be effective in depressed elderly patients. CBT has been particularly useful in those with partial response to antidepressant medications and in those elderly with diabetes, cardiac disorders and irritable bowel syndrome.

## PSYCHOSIS IN THE ELDERLY

Schizophrenia is traditionally considered as the disorder of the young adults (second or third decade of life). However, it has been found that 23% of the schizophrenia occurs in adults above 40 yrs and 3% in those above 60 yrs. Kraepelin found a group of subjects with symptoms characterized by a cognitive decline with hallucinations and delusions, without any negative symptoms such as emotional dullness or loss of volition; similar to those of dementia praecox and initially coined a term called 'Paraphrenia'. Currently, schizophrenia and schizophrenia-like psychoses in the elderly can be divided as late-onset (40–60 years) schizophrenia and very-late-onset (over 60 years) schizophrenia-like psychoses. However, late onset psychosis is not present in ICD-10 or DSM-IV. It is very common in females and the female to male ratio ranges from 4:1 to 20: 1. Usually they have sensory impairments such as deafness and visual impairment.

The psychotic symptoms include hallucinations, delusions and affective symptoms. Hallucinations may include simple auditory, auditory commenting type (derogatory or passing remarks on their actions), visual type (esp. in those with visual impairment resembling Charles Bonnet syndrome) and other types such as olfactory, gustatory, and tactile hallucinations may also be present. Delusions include themes such as persecutory, theft, reference, control; at times grandiose and hypochondrical delusions also may be present. Partition-delusions are false beliefs that people, animals, material, or radiation can pass through a structure that would normally constitute a barrier (the door, ceiling, walls, or floor of a patient's home) to such passage and the source of intrusion is usually a neighbouring residence. It is commonly found in very-late-onset schizophrenia-like patients. Formal thought disorder are seen only in a few and thought alienation phenomenon and negative symptoms are not frequently seen. Depressive symptoms can also be present.

Psychotic symptoms can occur as part of other medical conditions such as delirium, dementia and affective disorders.

Psychosis can be sometimes produce by disorders of the brain such as stroke, tumour, Wilson disease, epilepsy; medical conditions such as vitamin $B_{12}$ deficiency, hepatic encephalopathy, uremia, acute intermittent porphyria, thyroid and adrenal disorders, etc); due to medications like corticosteroids, dopaminergic drugs (e.g. L-dopa, amantadine), interferons, stimulants, anticholinergics (trihexiphenidyl) and rarely with antiarrhythmics, digitalis, anesthetics, antimalarial drugs (mefloquine), antituberculous drugs (D-cycloserine, ethambutol, isoniazid), antibiotics (ciprofloxacin), antivirals (efavirenz, acyclovir) antineoplastics (ifosfamide) and drugs of abuse such as alcohol, sedative-hypnotics, and recreational drugs.

The management involves evaluation of any treatment causes as mentioned above and the treatment of the primary disorder. Neuroimaging is very important in late onset psychosis.

The pharmacological management includes low dose of FGAs or SGAs antipsychotics. Research studies did not find any significant differences in the efficacy of the antipsychotics but there side-effect profiles were different. SGAs can cause stroke and metabolic syndrome (such as obesity, glucose intolerance, new onset of type 2 DM, diabetic ketoacidosis and dyslipidaemia). The FGAs can cause extrapyramidal syndrome and tardive dyskinesia. Pharmacological treatments have to be formulated based on case by case basis. Low dose risperidone has been recommended by experts as the first line treatment in late-life schizophrenia. Quetiapine (100 to 300 mg/day), olanzapine (2.5 to 10 mg/day) and aripiprazole (5–15 mg/day) have been recommended as second line of treatment. Low dose haloperidol also has been found to be useful in patients with cardiac disorders and metabolic syndrome. It also has an advantage; that it can be given in parenteral form for patients who are agitated. Psychosocial treatments such as psychoeducation, CBT, social skills training, problem solving techniques and compensatory aids for neurocognitive impairments are helpful in them.

| Table 11.4: Differences between delirium and dementia | | |
|---|---|---|
| Features | Delirium | Dementia |
| Onset | Abrupt | Subacute or insidious |
| Course | Fluctuates hourly, lucid periods in a day, confusion worsens at night or on sensory deprivation | Chronic; progresses gradually |
| Duration | Days to months; usually reversible | Months to years; Progressive and irreversible; Progresses to death |
| Consciousness | Clouding and confusion | Clear initially but can worsen in the late stages with delirium |
| Hallucinations | Usually visual, auditory and illusions present | Depends on the type of dementia, early presentation of hallucinations (diffuse Lewy body dementia) or later stages of Alzheimer's dementia |
| Delusions | Fleeting | Often absent |
| Attention/ concentration | Impaired normal | Initially normal but impaired in late stages |
| Memory | Significant impairment | Depending on the type of dementia, memory impairment can be initial or later |
| Psychomotor | Increased, reduced or shifting unpredictably | Often normal but with once behavioural problems sets in can worsen |
| Speech | Often incoherent | Usually coherent untillate stage |
| Thinking | Incoherent | Restricted and worsens in the later stages |

Contd.

**Table 11.4:** Differences between delirium and dementia (Contd.)

| Features | Delirium | Dementia |
|---|---|---|
| Sleep/wake cycle | Disturbed; changes hourly reversal | Disturbed; day/night |
| Causes | Post-traumatic, postictal, alcohol withdrawal, infections, metabolic (hyponatremia, hypoglycemia) and constipation | Degenerative process |

**Table 11.5:** Differences between pseudodementia and dementia

| | Depression (pseudo-dementia) | Dementia |
|---|---|---|
| 1. | Onset precisely outlined | Imprecise |
| 2. | Symptoms of short duration and rapid progression | Insidious onset and gradually progressive |
| 3. 4. | Disabilities highlighted Quick to give up questions and a little effort to perform tasks, but persists with encouragement | Disabilities concealed Struggles with performance of the task and fails |
| 5. | Frequently gives "Don't know" answers | Near miss answers |
| 6. | Cognitive functions fluctuates and behaviour is incongruent with the cognitive dysfunction | Stable and worsening |
| 7. | Outperformed categorical fluency task (i.e. "animals"). | Did not do well in categorical fluency task |
| 8. | Memory dysfunctions are of recent events and remote and improves with treatment of depressive disorders | Memory dysfunctions initially are mainly recent and does not improve |

Contd.

**Table 11.5:** Differences between pseudodementia and dementia
(Contd.)

| | Depression (pseudo-dementia) | Dementia |
|---|---|---|
| 9. | Less rapid rate of forgetting | More rapid rate of forgetting |
| 10. | Memory gaps for special period or events common | Unusual |
| 11. | Neurological defects (aphasia, apraxia, agnosias) often not present | Neurological defects often present |
| 12. | Usually communicates a strong sense of distress and affective changes are prominent | Often appears unconcerned with labile and shallow affect |

## REFERENCES/FURTHER READING

1. Anthony S. David, Simon Fleminger, Michael D. Kopelman, Simon Lovestone, John D.C. Mellers (Eds.). (2009). Lishman's Organic Psychiatry: A Textbook of Neuropsychiatry.

2. Blazer, D. G., and Steffens, D. C. (Eds.). (2010). The American psychiatric publishing textbook of geriatric psychiatry. American Psychiatric Pub.

3. Craig Gordon C and Martin J D. Mild cognitive impairment. (2013). Expert Rev. Neurother. 13(11), 1247–1261.

4. Cummings, J. L., Isaacson, R. S., Schmitt, F. A., and Velting, D. M. (2015). A practical algorithm for managing Alzheimer's disease: what, when, and why? Annals of Clinical and Translational Neurology.

5. Grover, S., and Kate, N. (2012). Assessment scales for delirium: A review. World Journal of Psychiatry, 2(4), 58.

6. JiniGopinath and Johnson Pradeep. R (Eds.). (2013) Essentials of Psychiatric Interviewing and Mental Status Examination. Vol 1, Cosmos Printers and Publishers. Bangalore.

7. Kaplan and Sadock's Synopsis of Psychiatry: Behavioral Sciences/ Clinical Psychiatry Paperback. Benjamin J. Sadock (Author), Virginia A. Sadock (Author), Dr. Pedro Ruiz MD (Author). 11th ed., 2014.

8. New Oxford Textbook of Psychiatry. Edited by Michael Gelder, Nancy Andreasen, Juan Lopez-Ibor, and John Geddes. 2nd ed., Oxford University Press, 2012

9. Organic Mental Disorders. Kalyanasundaram, Johnson Pradeep.R. Essentials of Postgraduate Psychiatry. Authors. J.N. Vyas, Shree Ram Ghimire, NK Bohra, Neena Bohra, VK Razdan, Hemant Vyas, MaridulaPurohit. 2nd Edition. 2015. Paras Medical Publishers, ISBN: 9788181914316.

10. S. Siva Raju. 2011. "Studies on Ageing in India: A Review", BKPAI Working Paper No. 2, United Nations Population Fund (UNFPA), New

11. Strub RL, Black FW. The Mental Status Examination in Neurology, 4th ed, FA Davis, Philadelphia 2000.

# 12

# Examination of Stuporous and Uncooperative Patients

S Rajkumar

Any young doctor attached to a neuro-psychiatric service or an emergency casualty department, would do well to ask 'within' himself three basic though arbitrary questions concerning the patient:

1. Is the patient predominantly 'normal' or 'abnormal'?
2. Is the abnormality predominantly of organic or psychogenic origin?
3. Is the psychiatric condition predominantly psychotic or neurotic?

Theoretical discussion in standard textbooks do dilute these differences but much progressive steps in examination could go a long way in diagnosing the disorder faster, prevent mistakes and avoid unnecessary laboratory investigations.

One should be cautious in: (a) not missing early signs of organic impairment, (b) being aware that nothing prevents a patient with functional illness from developing a neurological or systemic disorder.

Readers should supplement the following information with that from chapters on 'Neurological Assessment of Psychiatry Patients' and 'Primary Mental Functions'.

## CONSCIOUSNESS

Consciousness means awareness of self and environment. Its precise limits are extremely hard to define satisfactorily. However, there are two aspects of consciousness, and different types and distributions of brain disease affect them differently.

**203**

One is the content of consciousness, the sum of mental functions. The other is arousal, which behaviourally at least is closely linked with the appearance of wakefulness. The content of consciousness is largely the function of the cerebral hemispheres and the arousal part of consciousness, that of brainstem structures (the diencephalon, midbrain and pons).

Stupor is unresponsiveness from which the subject can be aroused only by vigorous and repeated stimuli. Coma is a unarousable unresponsiveness. It is not always easy to determine whether or not a patient is in coma, and even more so when one has to differentiate coma-like states due to organic cerebral dysfunction from psychogenic causes such as catatonic, depressive or hysterical stupor.

**The clinical approach to stuporous patients**

1. History
2. Physical Examination
   A. General
      a. Cardiovascular—Heart rate and BP
      b. Respiratory—Respirations: Rate, type
      c. Nuchal tone
      d. Body temperature
      e. General examination
   B. Neurological
      a. Fundoscopic examination
      b. Eye position and movements
      c. Pupils: Size and reaction
      d. Movements and reflex activity
      e. Muscle tone and posture
      f. Motor power
3. Laboratory Screening
   a. Urine
   b. Blood
   c. Spinal fluid

d. X-ray

e. EEG

f. Computerized Axial Tomography

The time lapse from the onset of the unconsciousness is an important consideration which should be specifically noted; e.g. convulsions as a cause of unconsciousness rarely last beyond 15 minutes, and while there may be postictal confusion lasting at times for hours, this invariably clears, rather than deepens, as a function of time. In contrast, certain types of injury, e.g. extradural or subdural haemorrhages, usually get worse after an initial lucid period, rapidly in the case of extradural bleeding and more gradually in subdural haematoma. The difference in the rapidity of developing unconsciousness in the natural history of these conditions is the result of the different haemorrhagic pressures; the extradural haemorrhage being under arterial and the subdural under venous pressure levels in most instances.

The history may also quickly alert the examiner to a subsequent convenient and pragmatic differentiation, i.e. unconsciousness with neurologic signs and symptoms in contrast to that without such signs.

A patient whose loss of consciousness is preceded historically by neurologic signs or symptoms, such as the presence of convulsions, confusion, hallucinations or severe headache, or any focal complaint, such as diplopia, vertigo numbness, weakness, or ataxia must be considered to have a disease affecting the central nervous system directly. On the other hand, unconsciousness without premonitory central nervous system signs most likely will be the result of diseases of other systems affecting the central nervous system secondarily or, at least, likely to be cerebro-toxic or metabolic in origin in which the nervous system is directly and at times exclusively, affected. There are, of course, many occasions in which signs of disease of the central nervous system, while present, may be obscure enough to be missed.

Although more details on neurological examination are elaborated in another chapter, it is outlined here in view of its importance.

We have had a few instances in which a diagnosis has been missed badly.

## Illustration I

A middle-aged woman, who used to get 'trance' attacks, was one day brought to the psychiatric outpatient department in a stuporous state. Clinically a diagnosis of 'hysterical reaction' was made and she was started on Trimipramine 25 mg at bedtime, in view of depressive features. Two days later she was brought in the same slate and assessed by neurologist and the same diagnosis confirmed. A week later she developed other features indicating a slowly progressive meningioma in the frontal region.

## Illustration 2

A high school student from Andamans had a 'Schizophrenic Reaction' for which he was treated with antipsychotic drugs and he improved well. Nine months later he came for review to Madras (and was found to have improved considerably). We maintained him on trifluoperazine 5 mg daily. Three days later he returned to Andamans, and strangely, he could not walk down from the aeroplane in Port Blair. A physician there diagnosed the condition to be 'Eskazine Drug Reaction' and stopped the drug. Within three days he developed further weakness in the limbs necessitating his contacting us. It was actually a case of acute infective polyneuritis. (Guillain-Barré syndrome).

The lesson is that nothing prevents a hysterical or schizophrenic patient from developing a space occupying lesion or an acute infection. Missing such diagnosis would be catastrophic.

Returning to the question of normality vs abnormality with reference to stuporous states, one should exclude the condition of malingering, which is an extremely rare condition. 'Malingering' is a wilful, deliberate, fraudulent imitation or exaggeration of illness, usually intended to deceive others, and under most circumstances, conceived for the purpose of gaining a consciously desired end. In this state, the individual is defensive, hostile, and refuses or resists frequent examinations quite unlike the hysterical patient. The diagnosis of hysteria in an unconscious patient "often tells more about the physician's lack of knowledge than the patient's disease" has been amply documented.

Psychogenic unresponsiveness sustained for more than a few minutes is uncommon. It was the final diagnosis in only 4 of the original 386 stuporous patients encountered by Plum and Posner in Chicago.

On the other hand, Joyston-Bechal (1966) examined the records of one hundred cases of stupor diagnosed at the Bethlem Royal and Maudsley Hospitals in order to obtain an indication of the frequency of different causes. Interestingly of the 100 cases, only 20 had stupor of organic origin and 14 could not be diagnosed with certainty.

Hysterical stupor is unconsciously determined, often influenced by suggestion, and there is a nonverbal communication. Often one notices what is termed 'secondary gain' in terms of sympathy and concern from relatives and others.

Any condition in which an organic cause for coma cannot be ferreted out, cannot be labelled as hysterical, unless the above features in terms of motive and intent, symptom pattern, and premorbid personality traits are assessed.

Very often these patients lie with their eyes closed, not attending to their surroundings. The pupils are equal and reactive, though the respiratory rate may alter. There is often active resistance to opening the eyelids, and they usually close rapidly when they are released. These patients offer no resistance to passive movements of the extremities although normal tone is present, and if an extremity is moved suddenly there may be momentary resistance. The deep tendon reflexes are usually normal, but they can be voluntarily suppressed and thus may be absent. The EEC is that of an awake patient rather than one in coma.

Catatonic stupor is often more difficult to differentiate from 'organic' unresponsiveness than hysteria or malingering outlined above. In catatonia, we see more often a semistuporous state, at times accompanied by autonomic abnormalities. Such a patient manifests extreme negativism, volitional and conative disturbances. The patient in catatonic stupor appears unresponsive to his environment but usually maintains consciousness and cognitive functions. This is substantiated by a normal neurological examination and an ability to recall events that took place during the stuporous state, after some recovery. The other features described in standard textbooks are oily skin, posturing (waxy flexibility), acrocyanosis, increased salivation, 'psychological pillow' and so on.

Depressive stupor is a condition which is often difficult to demarcate from other functional stupors as organic, catatonic, and hysterical stupors. A careful history into the antecedents, precipitating features/qualitative changes in mood, depressed facies (often with tears in eyes), suicidal ruminations, diurnal variations in mood and psycho-motor changes would assist the doctor in making a diagnosis.

## EXAMINATION OF THE UNCOOPERATIVE PATIENTS

In psychiatry one has to base the diagnosis largely on symptoms elicited rather than on 'signs'. In a uncooperative patient nonverbal communication needs to be recorded carefully, and at times the patient has to be observed on more than one occasion.

The best description on examination of uncooperative patients, apart from the issue raised above, is by Kirby (1921), as outlined by Mayer-Gross (1969). Lishman (1978) suggests the following format:

To what extent does the patient dress, feed himself or co-operate with feeding, attend to matters of hygiene and elimination?

Are the eyes open or shut? If open, are they apparently watchful and do they follow moving objects? If shut, do they open in response to stimulation, and is there resistance to passive opening?

Assess his response to graded stimulation. When aroused, does he become briefly alert and verbally responsive?

Is the physical posture comfortable, constrained, awkward, bizarre, or in any way indicative of possible delusional beliefs? Does the patient resume a previous posture if moved or when placed in an awkward or uncomfortable position? If so are movements meaningful? Do acts display special meaning, for example, on a possible delusional basis or in response to possible hallucinatory experiences?

Is the facial expression constant or varying, alert or vacant, blank or meaningful? Is it secretive, withdrawn, indicative of sadness, hopelessness or ecstasy? Does it betray attention to hallucinatory experiences? Is there any physical or emotional reaction to what is said or done to the patient, or within his hearing? Does he show an emotional response when sensitive subjects are discussed? Does he show signs of irritation or annoyance when moved against his wishes?

Examine the state of the musculature. Is it relaxed or rigid? Is rigidity increased by passive movements? Examine for negativism, flexibilities cerea, automatic obedience, echopraxia. Note evidence of resistiveness, irritability or defensive movements during examination.

In the neurological examination pay special attention to evidence of raised intracerebral pressure or diencephalic or upper brain stem disturbance, thus examine for papilloedema, observe equality and reactivity of pupils, note quality of respiration, look for evidence of long tract deficit in the limbs; and test for conjugate reflex eye movements on passive head rotation.

After recovery, examine for memory of events occurring during the abnormal phase, and for fantasies or other subjective experience occurring at the time.

With regard to 'Mutism', a condition in which the person does not speak and makes no attempt at spoken communication despite preservation of an adequate level of consciousness, the relevant questions are:

Is it elective, confined to some situations, or in relation to some persons but not others? Is the patient himself disturbed by it as shown by gesticulations or evidence of distress? Does he attempt to communicate by signs? On offering paper and pen, does he communicate in writing?

Distinguish mutism from severe motor dysphasia, dysarthria, aphonia, poverty of speech, and severe psychomotor retardation: Is partial vocalisation preserved? Are emotional ejaculations possible? Can simple 'Yes-no' answers be given? Test separately for ability to articulate (to whisper or make the lip movements of speech) and ability to phonate (to produce coarse vocalisations or to hum). Can he cough? Does he speak very occasionally and briefly on restricted themes? Does he reply or signal responses to some questions but only after a long delay?

A careful history from informants may sometimes enable distinctions to be made more readily than from examination alone.

## FURTHER READING

1. Joyston-Bechal MP. The Clinical Features and Outcome of Stupor. Br. J Psychiat 1996; 112: 967–981.

2. Lishman WA. Organic Psychiatry. The Psychological Consequences of Cerebral Disorder. Blackwell Scientific Publication, Oxford, 1978.

3. Meyer-Gross, Slater Roth. Clinical Psychiatry. Bailliere, Tindall and Cassell, London, 1966.

4. Mayo Clinic and Mayo Foundation. Clinical Examination in Neurology, 5th ed. Saunders, London, 1981.

5. Plum F, Posner JB. Diagnosis of Stupor and Coma, 2nd ed. Contemporary Neurological Series. Davis, Philadelphia, 1976.

6. The Dept. of Psychiatry Teaching Committee. The Institute of Psychiatry, London. Notes on Eliciting and Recording Clinical Information. Oxford University Press, 1973.

# 13

# Patients Posing Special Problems

James T Antony

Even for experienced clinical psychiatrists patients posing special problems create challenging situations. For a trainee psychiatrist these patients may sometimes generate a very high degree of personal anxiety. On occasions, an early encounter with a problem-patient, handled in a clumsy manner, makes the young doctor give up the choice of psychiatry as his field of specialisation.

An immediate task for a fresh trainee in any field of medicine is to master right clinical methods. If contact or encounter with patients—routine as well as those posing special problems—is to be effective and useful one must be proficient in clinical methods.

Psychiatry does not have a tradition to follow textbooks on the subject of clinical methods. To a certain extent this could be considered an advantage. Powdermaker (1948) was highly critical of the "Obsessive and mechanical use of a guide". She recommended a seminar method for learning clinical methods in psychiatry. While admitting the importance of fact-gathering, Powdermaker emphasised that "it is only when the patient senses that the doctor is a therapist rather than a fact-gatherer, there is some reduction in the patient's resistance and a real improvement in the doctor–patient relationship". A patient-orientation rather than a 'disease-orientation', is to be the mind-set.

The lack of proper textbooks and teaching aids is not the only reason for our present day backwardness in clinical skills in psychiatry. An equally important factor is our tendency to

**211**

fill up the gaps in our knowledge by applying whatever clinical methods we have learned from medicine as well as other fields. These methods essentially have a diagnostic orientation. There is a set sequence for history and clinical examination. In the end it must lead to a definite diagnosis. The emphasis is in not allowing patients to drift away or drag on too long with their sob-stories. The sequence to be followed to elicit findings is also clearly laid down—inspection, palpation and so on.

The time old method of medicine has been accepted by most specialities with some alterations and additions as regards to certain details. In psychiatry too, in the absence of a clearly laid down clinical approach, the traditional method of medicine provides the general format. Indeed, this approach has some advantages. For one thing it ensures that no important findings are missed. A more important point is that it satisfies the busy modern doctor who wants to finish with his examination of a patient in a 'reasonable' period of time. The overemphasis given to diagnosis in medical education these days may be another factor for doctors to be too pre-occupied about fact-gathering and being insistent on eliciting definite signs. A further reason is the naive belief that if diagnosis does not emerge with a standard history-taking and clinical examination, investigations are the answer. Our faith in technology is so supreme these days. The prevalent notion among some clinicians seems to be that given the right kind of equipment all diagnostic riddles can be solved in laboratories. It is unfashionable to think that if a diagnosis could not be made, one must go for more detailed interviews with the patient as well as significant persons in his life.

It is not that a diagnosis-orientation in psychiatry has been altogether discouraged by authorities. Slater and Roth (1969) stated that "if treatment is to be begun when it has best chance of success, a provisional diagnosis at least should be reached within the first week after the patient's admission". It is important that a provisional diagnosis is made at the earliest.

But the point is that one should not convey an impression that we are interested only in the patient's symptoms and not in him as a person. The useful dictum, in this regard has been given to us by Adolf Meyer who stated "We don't label our patients in this clinic, we try to understand them".

Painstaking and sometimes very lengthy interviews with patients and others is the only way, in many instances, to understand and diagnose—in the real sense of the term—sychiatric patients. Even on occasions when patients are apparently disturbed and noncooperative, the doctor must accept him as a human being entitled for a dignified treatment. He should be given due respect and has to be listened. Whatever reasonable demands that he may make must be allowed. To understand a patient properly, the mere content of his talk is not enough. The prosody-tone of voice, the inflection, the recognition of emotionally charged material and the meaning of silences are all important.

The actual techniques of conducting an interview is not being gone into here. But certain general points are worth mentioning. It is important to be very careful about elementary courtesies—like offering a proper seat for the patient, respecting his need for privacy, providing forthright and frank explanations to him regarding the doctor's proposed actions and so on. One more point, which I believe doctors cannot afford to forget is, that just as a doctor keeps on trying to diagnose and understand his patient, the patient too is constantly trying to 'diagnose' his doctor. A patient wants his doctor to be first and foremost, a sincere person. The second important thing a patient wants in his doctor is knowledge of his subject. It is always better for us to honestly measure up these expectations rather than just keep on pretending to be sincere and knowledgeable.

With these general considerations let us now examine some special points regarding certain types of patients, while keeping in mind that it is generally undesirable to 'type' patients, rather than trying to understand them as unique individuals.

## BOISTEROUS PATIENTS

Boisterous patients are in certain respects like angry children. They must be dealt with in a warm, kind and understanding manner. At the same time firmness and consistency are also important attributes.

A frequent cause for boisterousness and excitement is patient's perception of an arbitrary behaviour on the part of people around him as insulting. When the doctor hearing to his patient, before bystanders are allowed to give their version of the story, an excited patient will cool down and even leave it to the doctor to take suitable decision on his behalf.

Even with a warm, firm and receptive attitude of the doctor, an excited patient may need adequate tranquilization. Chlorpromazine intramuscular, or Haloperidol intravenous gives satisfactory results in most instances. There are occasions when physical restraint has to be used to control potentially violent behaviours. When a decision on application of restraint is taken it is important that the doctor does not desert his patient. He must provide leadership in handling this crisis situation, and also explain to the patient about the injection and also about the need to use restraints. It will be a good practice for doctors to review their physically-restrained patients every ten or fifteen minutes.

The general approach outlined above is applicable to most excited patients—schizophrenia, mania as well as organic psychoses. On the other hand, in an acute psychotic excitement with devastating overall disorganization of personality and also history of a strong precipitating factor (like a woman who broke down after witnessing the dastardly murder of her husband) the treatment aim must be to achieve immediate heavy sedation. A combination of Chlorpromazine and a barbiturate will be quite satisfactory. Any attempt to verbally communicate with such patients in the acute phase is futile. Detailed interview must wait till their disorganization has settled down completely.

One more instance where detailed interview and assessment of a patient has to wait is an excited and violent behaviour of epilepsy, both in postictal and psychomotor fits. Drug treatment sometimes combined with physical restraint is the immediate need in these patients, to protect themselves as well as others.

## PARANOID AND HOSTILE PATIENTS

Sometimes we meet relatives who find it very convenient "to tell patients that they are being taken to an old friend who has promised to solve their current legal problem. They are keen to persuade the doctor also to conceal his real identity. The relatives' version usually is that the moment patient finds out that he is with a psychiatrist there will be a violent explosion. But experience with these patients all along has shown that reality is exactly the opposite. A patient who wants to know the doctor's identity probably knows that already. It will be a serious mistake for a doctor to attempt deception. On the contrary, by being frank and sincere the doctor wins the patient's confidence and respect. Even when a patient asks such sensitive questions like "doctor, do you think that I have some mental illness"? the doctor should not give a misleading answer. His duty is to present the reality in the least traumatic manner and probably adding it up with warm reassurance.

Among paranoid and hostile patients a small proportion seems to have 'homosexual panic'. Such patients might be controlled easily by a doctor or nurse belonging to the opposite sex, though they are very hostile to doctors of the same sex. This sometimes is a useful point in their management. Also it has been reported that patients with 'latent homosexuality' may go to a panic state, when an injection is attempted. Probably the symbolic connotation of an injection is the reason. In such instances administration of drugs by oral route will be advisable.

## WITHDRAWN PATIENTS

The old, worn-out, diagnosis-oriented and fact-gathering approach is particularly unsuitable to deal with withdrawn patients. These patients, both schizophrenics as well as schizoid personalities, are persons who value their privacy very much. The doctor's eager questioning is viewed as unwelcome intrusions to their precious inner territories. The doctor who is always busy (and rather proud of this fact) is apt to get irritated and angry with his patient who is reluctant to communicate. He may sometimes be tempted to ask these patients an unfortunate question like "if you don't come out with facts, how do you expect me to help you"? It is indeed wrong for doctors to imagine that withdrawn patients will open-up by a volley of questions. Being autobiographical or a display of jocularity or even temper on the part of the doctor are all measures that would only damage doctor–patient relationship.

In his contact with withdrawn patients the doctor has to reduce his pace, so that both are tuned to the same wavelength. The interview may sometimes come to an uncomfortable halt. On such occasions it is for the doctor to wait on patiently. This tells the patient very effectively, though non-verbally, that "I understand your problems are of a very delicate nature". The doctor who is not impatient or inquisitive, does not pass a moral judgement on his patient's deeds and attitudes, but at the same time is warm and understanding, will eventually make a withdrawn patient trust him and come out with useful material from the history as well as his mental life.

The above points are valid while assessing mental status and the family situation of a withdrawn patient as well as in planning a therapeutic atmosphere for him in the hospital. A family where some members are too inquisitive, emotional and interfering, makes a withdrawn person worse. Similarly a hospital atmosphere that has too many social activities makes withdrawn patients upset. Attempts to improve the social skills of withdrawn patients without taking into account their need for privacy is unlikely to succeed.

## ANXIOUS PATIENTS

Anxious patients are keen to believe that their doctor has extra-ordinary knowledge, skill and goodness. At least some doctors are willing to play the role of a demigod. This indeed is a sick situation. The anxious patient is eager and ready to cling to his doctor, and the 'demigod doctor' enjoys his role of an eternal mother!

The above relationship is mutually satisfying. The patient finds a new sense of security with someone who has ready answers for all his day-to-day problems. For the doctor the boost for his ego works like a soft intoxicant. And more than this, the material benefits that the doctor can derive by such a faulty relationship is quite tempting.

The prevalence of the above malady is probably universal. One reason is that there are many built-in adverse factors that originate from present day economic and social systems and may be, are beyond the scope of individual doctors to correct.

It is important that doctors sometime introspect and analyse the scope and limitation of doctor–patient relationship, as regard to anxious patients. A doctor's role is only that of a doctor, nothing more, and of course nothing less. A lot of tact and diligence is needed to nurture such a doctor–patient relationship. Firmness and warmth are of equal importance. Even at the very first interview the doctor must have a clear view that one of his primary therapeutic aims is to make the patient self-reliant and independent of our caregiving medical system. At the same time he must not be reluctant to provide support, sometimes for a prolonged period, to a patient who really needs that.

## MANIPULATIVE PATIENTS

In the case of 'manipulative patients' doctors often take an attitude diametrically opposite to the one they have for anxious patients. They overtly neglect their manipulative patients. Even the term 'manipulative' has a pejorative sense. The implication of the term is that these patients are wilfully trying to take advantage of our system. 'Attention-seeking' is another term we use to denote these patients. And when we say 'attention seeking' it is implied that they are not 'attention-needing'. The net result is that once a patient acquires the label 'manipulative' in a hospital, everybody, doctor, nurse and attendant, treat him as an outcast. A sort of retaliative manipulative behaviour starts on the part of the medical establishment to drive the patient away.

It is important to be aware that most of these 'manipulative patients' are persons in serious distress-states. As such it has to be understood as an effort on their part to communicate their feelings to the relatives and doctor. A close look will convince the doctor that there is much in common between an anxious patient and a manipulative patient and therefore it is logical that both are treated with the same kind of balanced concern and warmth. The guideline should be that our attention to the patient's complaints should not reinforce or strengthen those symptoms; in the same way our rejection and dismissal of particular complaints should not give the impression that we are rejecting the patient altogether.

## SOMATISING PATIENTS

Somatising patients often have very complex reasons for developing a particular psycho-physiological reaction. The points mentioned in discussing anxious and manipulative patients are generally applicable here as well. There will not be much difficulty in dealing with these patients if only one has his concept of psychosomatics right. But a tendency to divide 'psyche' and 'soma' as though they are two separate territories is quite prevalent. Added to this there is a value-judgement in this area viewing anything somatic as 'real' and needing sympathy and understanding, whereas anything 'psychological' or 'functional' is 'unreal' and as such does not deserve any sympathy. The fact is that both 'psyche' and 'soma' or 'physical' and 'mental' are only two views of the same unitary reality.

Patients with 'somatisation' and patients with an 'organic lesion' deserve the same sympathetic understanding from the doctor. Concepts of aetiology are there for doctors to improve their ability to take better care of patients, and not to justify tough and cold positions against them.

## DEPRESSIVE PATIENTS

Depressive disorders are among the most common illnesses affecting humankind. Vast majority of depressives remain undiagnosed in the community, as they fail to recognise that they have a treatable disease. Even those depressives consulting doctors, the majority are not diagnosed. This may seem to be a paradox, with all our present day refinements in diagnostic criteria.

Depressed mood continues to be the central, predominant feature for diagnosing, whether it be major depressive disorder, dysthymic disorder or any other type of depressive disorder. And this depressed mood is something subjectively experienced by a patient and as such is not accessible to a doctor. What generally happens is that, when features usually associated with a depressed mood are elicited the presence of a depressed mood is assumed. This indeed is not a satisfactory state of things as a depressed mood even while it is present in the patient will not be picked by the doctor when his expected associated other features are absent. Another way a doctor could know about depressed mood is when the patient tells him about it. Indeed many patients do tell their doctor about their depressed mood. But for many patients, exposing their inner core emotional experience, even to their doctor is embarrassing, like stripping naked in the presence of total strangers.

By improving his rapport with patients there could be some progress, but even then a large proportion of patients fail to reveal their depressed mood.

The study of conscious experiences was emphasized by late 19th century philosophers and for this study they developed a field of knowledge named phenomenology. Karl Jaspers (1912) found that phenomenology is useful to clinical psychiatry, in that its methods are useful for a better understanding of patients' description of their conscious experiences.

**Jaspers gave three methods to determine what patients really experience.**

1. Immerse oneself, so to speak, in their gestures, behaviour, expressive movements.

2. Explore by direct questioning of the patients and by means of accounts they themselves, under our guidance, give of their experience.

3. Written self-descriptions.

It has been said by phenomenologists that some questions help one to come a little closer to what the patient has been experiencing in his conscious mind.

Questions like the following are quite useful in this regard. "How candid was the patient with himself?" "Or with me?"

"How adequate was his recognition of the mental phenomenon experienced by him?" "How suitable was his choice of words in describing them?"

"How correct was my understanding of his words?" Indeed all our known methods of science tell us that we are unable to transcend the frontiers of our consciousness and get to know the conscious experiences of our patients. But to elicit symptoms like depression one may realise often, that such an ability is needed.

Karl Jaspers' phenomenological methods certainly help us to be at least a little more close to our patients' experiential world. And integrating Jaspers' methods to our own clinical methods in psychiatry will go a long way to understand our patients better, especially those in painful predicaments like a depressed mood.

# 14 Child and Adolescent Psychiatry

Sitalakshmi George

## INTRODUCTION

Child and adolescent psychiatry has come a long way during the past few decades to be accepted as a separate branch of psychiatry. Many hospitals in India now have dedicated units to help children with mental health problems. Parents and teachers are increasingly concerned about children's academic and social progression; are able to identify problems in their behaviour or studies, and are seeking advice. As awareness has increased, there is increasing acceptance of child mental health services, and consequently a greater demand for such services.

A child is an individual with thoughts, emotions, interactions and relationships. Professionals need to reach the level of the child to understand their problems, to provide meaningful explanations, and to set down a plan of action to help the child and the family. A child grows rapidly so that its physical, mental and emotional needs also change rapidly. Health professionals should be aware of these changes so that we can make assessments appropriate to the current stage of development: Behaviours which are normal during a certain stage of development may be inappropriate during other stages.

To become a good child mental health professional, one has to be familiar with the stages of child development, level of intelligence, and skills to be achieved at each stage and educational needs of each stage. One should also be aware of psychosocial background of the families, family dynamics;

221

educational assessment and remedial education. There should be a good understanding of child intelligence assessment, parental assessment and type of parenting; and also a good knowledge of mental disorders in children and adults.

Assessment of children and adolescents takes time as many of these areas need to be covered, and information needs to be gathered from multiple sources (e.g. Parents, siblings, other relatives, school teachers and carers). The combined information and test results have to be interpreted before a diagnostic formulation can be arrived at, and a care plan put together.

### Stages of Development

There are many ways of assessing whether a child has achieved succeeding levels of development—often called milestones of development. At each milestone a child is expected to have achieved certain types of physical, intellectual and psychological skills. Using such milestones it is possible to ascertain whether development is adequate for that age, advanced for that age or whether the child is lagging behind. Development being a gradual and sometimes an uneven process, it is important to recognise that there can be overlaps between the stages, and temporary delays as well as quick corrections during development.

With these facts in mind, it is possible to describe the following stages in development.

1. Infancy (Birth – 2 years)

   This is a stage of rapid changes being influenced by prenatal, natal and postnatal events. It also becomes evident that there are many differences between babies—physical, tempe- ramental and physiological growth. There will be noticeable variations in the feeding and sleeping patterns. There will be rapid achievements of several milestones—from a totally helpless infant at birth to an independently walking and running two years old. Babies also begin to show 'stranger anxiety' starting around 4–6 months of age. This involves a natural moving away, or clinging and/or crying in the presence of unfamiliar people.

2. Preschool (2–4 years)

This is the stage when children become increasingly capable of eating and toileting. They may not become fully independent in these functions but learn to indicate these basic needs.

This is also the stage when children begin to attend playschool, giving them an opportunity to socialise with other children and adults, to observe and learn new social skills. They learn new words, their language skills moving from single words to two- or three-word sentences.

3. Early Childhood (4–8 years)

Children become independent in eating and toileting, and are ready for schooling. They are listening and learning new words; language skills are increasing; alphabets and numerals are introduced. Along with words and numbers, the child is also learning new behaviours, manners; beginning to distinguish right from wrong. Children need supervision, guidance and correction when they do wrong.

4. Late Childhood (8–12 years)

During this phase the child is becoming independent in activities of daily living like brushing teeth, bathing, and dressing. Sleep wake patterns become more settled. Child gets to practise good manners and behaviour. There is increasing mastery of reading, writing, spelling, and basic arithmetic.

5. Puberty (12–16 years)

The child progresses towards more physical and mental maturity, often with phases of rapid changes. While most children are able to accept these changes without much difficulty, such rapid changes can be overwhelming to many children. It is quite usual for children at this age to frequently check themselves out in the mirror or repeatedly ask for reassurance about their looks or appearance. By end of puberty children become independent in reading, writing and arithmetic.

6. Adolescence (12–18 years)

The age limits of adolescence vary in different cultures, some even accept adolescence up to 21 years of age. This is the period when an individual moves from dependence to independence in all areas. This is also the age when physical growth, psychosexual development and hormonal changes reach the final stages of development. Children face a lot of stress regarding educational achievements, choosing future studies/work, meeting parental aspirations and peer pressures.

Supportive parents, teachers and school counsellors can go a long way in shaping and nurturing the personality of the child during this critical phase of development. Most of the personality characteristics formed by this age, are relatively permanent and difficult to change in future.

## CLASSIFICATION

Classification is important in all branches of medicine to better understand a disorder, its natural course, treatment and prognosis; and to communicate with other professionals. Classification is more complex and difficult in the field of mental health for a number of reasons.

One of the first proponents of what later became known as Multiaxial Classification was Michael Rutter (1969). He emphasised that many children who attended child mental health services did not have a primary mental disorder. The consultation was for issues related to development, intelligence, physical illnesses the child suffered from, or social issues. He asserted that a complete assessment of a child should include all these areas, and the results of the assessment should specify whether the child had problems in any one, or all these areas.

Multiaxial Classification of Child and Adolescent Psychiatric Disorders of ICD 10 includes six Axes along which a child should be assessed.

Axis I covers clinical psychiatric syndromes (e.g. conduct disorder, tic disorder)

Axis II deals with specific disorders of psychological development (e.g. specific reading disorder)

Axis III describes the intellectual level (e.g. mild mental retardation)

Axis IV mentions any associated medical condition (e.g. cerebral palsy, bronchial asthma)

Axis V describes any associated abnormal psychosocial situations (e.g. family discord, acute life events)

Axis VI provides a global assessment of psychosocial disability (e.g. 'child has moderate social disability', or is 'unable to function in most areas')

## AXIS I

### CLINICAL PSYCHIATRIC SYNDROMES

Many of the disorders listed in the ICD which occur in adults, may also occur in children. The appropriate code is used to indicate the presence of such disorders in children. Conditions like depression, mania, obsessive compulsive disorder, substance misuse and related conditions are often encountered in children and adolescents.

The commonest childhood disorders in Axis I are grouped under the heading "Behavioural and Emotional Disorders with Onset Usually Occurring in Childhood and Adolescence" (F90 – F98). Some of the more prevalent conditions in this group are the following:

### HYPERKINETIC DISORDERS (F90.0–F90.1)

**F90.0 Disturbance of activity and attention:** This disorder usually begins before age 5 years, and is commonly referred to as attention deficit hyperactivity disorder (ADHD). The usual symptoms are inattention, impulsivity and hyperactivity; and the symptoms are present in more than one situation (e.g. home, classroom, playground). The condition is three times more common in boys than girls.

Assessment involves a detailed history including reports from school, and direct observation. Treatment of milder forms of ADHD involves limit setting and parent skills training. Moderate to severe cases need treatment with stimulant medication like methylphenidate or other medications like atomoxetine.

**F90.1 Hyperkinetic Conduct Disorder:** This condition will meet the criteria for both hyperkinetic disorder and conduct disorder.

## CONDUCT DISORDERS (F91.0–F91.3)

This group of disorders is characterised by repetitive dissocial, aggressive, defiant and disobedient behaviour. There may also be stealing, lying, temper tantrums, bullying, excessive quarrelling and fighting, destroying things, cruelty to animals and people, truancy and running away from home. Depending on certain characteristics, the condition may be divided into subgroups:

**F91.0 Conduct Disorder Confined to the Family Context** in which the disordered behaviour is entirely or almost entirely confined to the home and/or to interactions with members of the family or household

**F91.1 Un-socialised Conduct Disorder** is diagnosed when a child has conduct disorder with limited or poor peer relationships, evidenced by rejection by peers, being socially isolated and lacking close friends.

**F91.2 Socialised Conduct Disorder** is diagnosed when the child with conduct disorder is generally well integrated into their peer group, and has friends.

**F91.3 Oppositional Defiant Disorder** is generally diagnosed before the age of 9 or 10 years, and is defined by the presence of markedly defiant, disobedient, provocative behaviour. There is no severe dissocial or aggressive acts that violate the law or the rights of others.

**F92 Mixed Disorder of Conduct and Emotions:** It is characterised by aggressive, dissocial, defiant behaviour associated with depression, anxiety or emotional upsets.

Assessment of conduct disorder requires detailed descriptions of behaviour at home, school, and other settings.

Parent skills training alone can bring about dramatic changes in the child's behaviour. However, if the problem is moderate or severe, along with skills training for parents, the child may require short periods of medication to control aggression. Many clinicians use small doses of antipsychotics in such situations.

## F93: EMOTIONAL DISORDERS WITH ONSET SPECIFIC TO CHILDHOOD

### F93.0: Separation Anxiety Disorder of Childhood.

The child experiences fear of separating from or losing the major attachment figure. The child may express fears of being lost or kidnapped; or of being alone. There may be somatic symptoms like nausea, vomiting or headaches. Separation anxiety is often a cause of school refusal.

**F93.1 Phobic anxiety disorder of childhood:** It is characterised by fear of specific objects or situations

**F93.2 Social anxiety disorder of childhood:** It is a persistent fear and avoidance of strangers leading to significant impairment of social functioning. The child often clings to the parent or caregiver.

**F93.3 Sibling rivalry disorder:** It is denoted by jealousy or rivalry shown as marked competition for attention and affection. The child may also exhibit towards the sibling significant hostility and malice, avoid sharing things and have negative interactions.

Assessment of childhood emotional disorders requires the identification of anxiety or depression. The presentation of these may not be as evident as in adults, and the clinician needs to be aware of the ways children experience anxiety and depression. If there are significant factors in the environment leading to the emotional changes, these factors should be modified. If the symptoms cause a change in the child's temperament, or affect school performance and adjustments at home, anxiolytics or antidepressant medication should be considered.

## AXIS II

## DISORDERS OF PSYCHOLOGICAL DEVELOPMENT

## SPECIFIC DEVELOPMENTAL DISORDERS OF SPEECH AND LANGUAGE (F80.0–F80.2)

**F80.0 Specific speech articulation disorder:** It is a specific developmental disorder in which the child's use of speech sounds is below the appropriate level for the mental age; the child has a normal level of language skills

**F80.1 Expressive language disorder:** The child's ability to use expressive spoken language is markedly below the appropriate level for the mental age; language comprehension is within normal limits. There may or may not be articulation difficulties.

**F80.2 Receptive language disorder:** The child's understanding of language is below the appropriate level. This is usually associated with marked disturbance of expressive language and articulation.

A child with any of these speech or language disorder may be referred to a speech therapist who will be able to make the appropriate assessment and provide speech training.

## SPECIFIC DEVELOPMENTAL DISORDERS OF SCHOLASTIC SKILLS (F81.0–F81.2)

Scholastic skills like reading, writing or arithmetic may fail to develop in some children from the early stages of development. This is not simply a consequence of a lack of opportunity to learn; rather, this is the result of an underlying biological dysfunction. The impairment must be specific to the scholastic skill, and cannot be explained as part of general lack of intelligence, or inadequate teaching inputs.

**F81.0 Specific reading disorder:** This involves a specific impairment in the development of reading skills including reading comprehension, reading word recognition, oral reading and performance of tasks requiring reading.

**F81.1 Specific spelling disorder:** This is a specific impairment in the development of spelling skills in the absence of specific reading disorder. The ability to spell orally and to write out words correctly are *both* affected. The spelling errors tend to be predominantly phonetically accurate.

**F81.2 Specific disorder of arithmetical skills:** This impairment consists of deficits in basic computational skills of addition, subtraction, multiplication and division. The child may have difficulty to understand the concepts underlying particular arithmetical operations; lack of understanding of mathematical terms and signs, aligning numbers or inserting decimal points or symbols during calculations, and inability to learn multiplication tables satisfactorily.

A child with specific language or scholastic disorder will require a detailed assessment of the academic skills and an intelligence assessment to find out what level the child is functioning at. Depending on this the child can be provided appropriate guidance and remedial education. Many schools do provide such remedial teaching now.

## PERVASIVE DEVELOPMENTAL DISORDERS (F84.0–F84.5)

This group of disorders (PDD) is characterised by abnormalities in reciprocal social interactions, patterns of communication, and restricted, stereotyped and repetitive interests and activities.

**F84.0 Childhood autism:** Symptoms become apparent before 3 years age, often without any previous period of normal development. There is abnormal functioning in all three areas of social interaction, communication, and restricted, repetitive behaviour. The disorder is three to four times more common in boys than in girls. They are unable to appreciate social-emotional cues or to reciprocate them. Language skills may not develop, or there will be lack of social usage of whatever language skills are present. There is also restricted, repetitive behaviour, interests, and activities. There is a preference for routine in day to day functioning; there may be specific attachment to unusual objects, and the children may insist on particular routines/rituals of a non-functional character. All levels of intellectual functioning can occur, though there is significant mental retardation in three-fourths of cases.

**F84.1 Atypical autism:** This is diagnosed when the age of onset is beyond three years; or if there are insufficient abnormalities in one or two of the three areas described. Atypical autism is often diagnosed when pervasive developmental disorder occur in children with profound mental retardation.

**F84.2 Rett's syndrome:** Reported only in girls, onset of this condition usually occurs between 7 and 24 months of age, with an apparently normal or near normal development till then. This is followed by partial or complete loss of hand skills and speech, and slowing of head growth. Severe mental handicap, seizures, and abnormalities of trunk and spine also develop in most children with Rett's syndrome.

**F84.5 Asperger's syndrome:** There is no general delay in language or cognitive development, though there are characteristic abnormalities of social interaction together with restricted, repetitive interests and activities; and affected individuals are often clumsy. Most individuals are of normal intelligence. The condition occurs predominantly in boys; and at least some cases may be considered mild varieties of autism.

Management of pervasive developmental disorder begins with direct observation and detailed assessment of the child's behaviour. Much thinking needs to go into understand the meaning of a particular behaviour and to plan remedial measures. The clinician also needs to learn from the parents their understanding of the child's behaviour, and their attempts to cope with such behaviours. It will soon become apparent that each child is unique, and that the training schedules have to be individualised.

Starting training at the earliest is particularly important, and frequent changes need to be made in the training as the child progresses and matures. Different programmes may be needed for home, school and other settings.

Children with PDD are prone to anxiety, obsessive compulsive behaviour, psychosis and epilepsy. These conditions usually require the use of appropriate medications.

## AXIS III

## INTELLECTUAL LEVEL

## MENTAL RETARDATION (F70-F79)

Mental retardation is a condition of arrested or incomplete development of the mind, characterised by impairment of cognitive, language, motor, and social abilities. Retardation can occur with or without any other mental or physical disorder. Mentally retarded individuals are vulnerable to develop other mental disorders. In addition, they are at greater risk of exploitation and physical/sexual abuse.

**F70 Mild mental retardation:** Most people with mild mental retardation can use speech for everyday purposes, and most also achieve full independence in self-care, and in practical and domestic skills. However, academic school work is affected though many can be helped by specially designed education methods. Many individuals become capable of working especially in unskilled and semiskilled work. If assessed properly they are seen to fall into an IQ range of 50–69.

**F71 Moderate mental retardation:** Individuals in this category fall into IQ range of 35–49. Comprehension and use of language are limited; and achievement of self-care and motor skills is also impaired—some need supervision throughout life. Though such people are generally fully mobile, and physically active, complete independent living in adult life is rarely possible.

**F72 Severe mental retardation:** The IQ is usually in the range of 20–34. In addition to lower levels of achievements, most suffer from motor impairment or other associated deficits, indicating the presence of significant damage to or mal-development of the central nervous system.

**F73 Profound mental retardation:** Affected individuals are severely limited in their ability to understand or comply with requests or instructions. Most are severely restricted in mobility and require constant help and supervision; most are incontinent. IQ in this category is estimated to be under 20.

## AXIS IV

### MEDICAL CONDITIONS

This axis provides for coding of non-psychiatric medical conditions which are currently present. Such conditions should be coded even if they are not considered significant in the causation of the psychiatric condition. Acts of self-harm should also be recorded in Axis IV.

## AXIS V

### ASSOCIATED PSYCHOSOCIAL SITUATION

Any associated psychosocial situation involving the patient should be coded in this Axis. Such situations should be coded regardless of whether they are thought to have caused the psychiatric condition. It is important to recognise that any abnormal psychosocial situation will be a factor to be taken into consideration in therapeutic planning. There are a number of situations for which ICD codes are available and which are obviously important in both understanding the causation of the psychiatric condition and in care planning. Examples include 'Problems related to social environment' (Z60.0–Z60.8), 'Problems related to negative life events in childhood' (Z61.0–Z61.8), and 'Other problems related to upbringing' (Z62.0–Z62.8)

## AXIS VI

### GLOBAL ASSESSMENT OF PSYCHOSOCIAL DISABILITY

This axis reflects the patient's psychological, social and occupational functioning at the time of clinical assessment. The code entered reflects the examiner's assessment of the patient's disabilities in functioning as a consequence of psychiatric disorder, specific disorders of psychological development and/or mental retardation. There are nine levels of social functioning/disability—e.g. 'good social functioning' (code 0), 'moderate social disability' (code 3), or 'profound and pervasive social disability' (code 8).

## CONCLUSION

Child mental health services have made tremendous progress in India in the last 25 years, though there still are many areas with no access to such services. Much work—clinical and research—is being done in several centres across the country.

Awareness is spreading in the community, and in schools; and many schools have responded by providing guidance and counselling to children and parents.

New laws, and better implementation of laws are making a dent on child abuse and child labour and are improving opportunities for children's education.

It is being recognised that early intervention is fundamental to success in child mental health problems. Children grow rapidly, and need to acquire new skills appropriate to stages of development; if they are not able to do so, they find it difficult to acquire skills of the subsequent stages.

Finally, child mental health services are both therapeutic and preventive. Childhood intervention is uniquely positioned to achieve the twin aims of reducing the suffering of children who is experiencing a disorder; and of preventing the development of later mental and personality disorders.

## FURTHER READING

1. Diagnostic and Statistical Manual of Mental Disorders, Fifth Edition (2013): American Psychiatric Association.
2. Michael Rutter et al. (2014): Rutter's Child and Adolescent Psychiatry, 5th Edition, Wiley-Blackwell.
3. Molly McVoy et al (ed) 2013: Clinical Manual of Child and Adolescent Psychopharmacology, Second Edition, American Psychiatric Publishing.
4. The ICD–10 Classification of Mental and Behavioural Disorders. (1992): World Health Organization, Oxford University Press.

# 15

# Influence of Culture on the Phenomenology in Psychiatry

S Santhakumar, PM Vasudevan

## INTRODUCTION

There is a story about a renowned English Professor of Psychiatry who when asked by his students as to what books they should study for psychiatry, replied "The Bible, Aesop's, Fables, and Shakespeare". The message is quite clear. Psychiatry and other psychological sciences should have their roots in the particular culture.

Culture refers to the complex pattern of learnt behaviour, values, customs and beliefs, shared by members of a particular community. According to Rajaji it is "the sum total of the way of living built by groups of human beings and transmitted from one generation to another". "People each with their own long history build up separate patterns of culture. There is much that is common, but also a great deal that is particular to each nation". The study of psychiatry within the framework of these cultural peculiarities and similarities of different cultural setting is the subject matter of trans-cultural psychiatry. The culture implies many aspects of the ways of living: Physical setting or what the sociologists call the "Archefacts", social milieu or the "Socifacts" and the psychological make up of its population or "Mentifacts". All these aspects with their reciprocal interactions give rise to the particular cultural characteristic of a group. Just as a physical attribute like climate determines the mode of clothing of a population, the pattern of social set up, the customs, beliefs and attitudes influence the personality organisation of the individuals of a society. Culture influences the coping mechanisms of an individual and the patterns of response to stresses, both physical and psycho-social. Culture also to a considerable extent functions as an 'arbitrator' in delineating normal from abnormal behaviour. Certain things coming under normal beliefs and behaviours in a particular culture may be considered frankly abnormal in another. For example, it is not uncommon for many normal illiterates in our villages to attribute an illness or calamity to some black magic by his or her enemies, whereas this may strike as a frankly abnormal belief (delusion) to a westerner not conversant with our culture.

It is not an exaggeration to say that society sets guidelines as to how an individual should behave in response to different stresses or situations. Thus there are some organised ways for mourning and expressions of grief. Funeral processions with accompaniment of merry making and dances found in certain communities of South India will astonish somebody from an alien culture. The mode of expression of behavioural abnormality again is to a great extent influenced by culture. As Deveneux, a famous trans-cultural psychiatrist, has suggested the symptoms of a psychological disturbance tend to conform to the cultural expectation of how symptoms should appear.

Finally it is needless to say that the socio-cultural milieu plays a paramount role in our approach to management including rehabilitation of the psychiatrically ill. Culture dictates its members their conceptions of illness and its predispositions as well as its outcome. The culture in no small measure colours the symptoms with which patients present themselves for help.

## INFLUENCE OF CULTURE ON THE PHENOMENOLOGY OF PSYCHIATRIC ILLNESS

Till recently many western psychiatrists believed that mental illness is rare among many of the underdeveloped countries. That this is not the case has been established by many epidemiological studies in these countries as well as cross-cultural and trans-cultural studies. The WHO conducted multi-centred studies spread over different continents and countries on two of the major psychiatric diseases, namely schizophrenia and depression. These and the recent researches in these fields highlight the following facts:

1. Almost all types of mental illness are present in every part of the world.
2. While the core symptoms of a particular disease are met with in all cultures, there are many differences with respect to the manifest symptoms. These differences are attributable to what is called the 'pathoplastic' effect of the culture on the illness.
3. There are certain syndromes met with almost exclusively in certain cultures. These are called 'Culture Bound Syndromes'.

We will now examine a few of this 'pathoplastic' effects of our culture on some of the major psychiatric diseases.

## PSYCHOSES

### 1. Schizophrenia and Delusional Disorder

Like in other countries schizophrenia is a common psychotic illness in our population. It is a major form of mental illness which affects all aspects of the personality—cognitive, affective, and connective and leads to progressive deterioration in many cases.

Symptoms described in western textbooks are most often come across in our patients also. These include perceptual abnormalities like hallucinations, thought disorders like poverty of ideas, though it block, perseveration, thought withdrawal, thought insertion, thought broadcast and referential ideas, ideas of influence, passivity phenomena primary and secondary delusions, and in the affective sphere emotional blunting (total apathy in extreme cases), emotional incongruence or inappropriateness, as well as increased or decreased volitional (motor) activity. It is generally agreed that all First Rank Symptoms (FRS) of Schneider are met with as commonly in India as in western countries. However, the influence of our cultural milieu is evident from the contents of symptoms like hallucinations and delusions. Even among our population the educational status, religious beliefs, etc. also influence the contents of these symptoms. For example, it is not uncommon for many rural illiterate people to base their persecutory delusion on angry ancestors or black magic by relatives and in-laws through talisman ('Yanthram', 'thakidu'), etc. while the theme in an educated urban youth may be involvement of CBI, sophisticated mechanisms like computer, electronic devices, etc.

It is customary to sub-type schizophrenia into four major groups: Simple, Hebephrenic, Catatonic and Paranoid. Simple variety lacks florid symptoms and such patients are not usually brought for consultation. There is a gradual deterioration in personality in them, many of them ending up as beggars, prostitutes and criminals. Hebephrenic type usually commences at adolescent stage and shows gross emotional blunting and incongruity. The leading symptoms in catatonic schizophrenia are usually volitional, manifesting either as catatonic excitement or stupor. Paranoid type usually starts later in life and its clinical picture is typically characterised by delusions of persecution. The international pilot study of schizophrenia found that in India schizophrenia had a large proportion, of catatonic features but other types of schizophrenia are also quite common.

Wittkover and Rin have observed that the predominance of catatonic symptoms is due to the eastern ways of life which is "rigidly hierarchical and formal, and prizes and rewards introversion; the frequency of catatonic states in India are due to India's traditional tendency to reject society, and the postures adopted by certain types of sanyasins or yogis."

'Persistent delusional disorders' form a heterogeneous group characterised by presence of long standing delusions. The culture dictates the theme of the delusions.

## 2. Affective Disorders

Recent studies have been able to refute the earlier contention that manic-depressive psychosis and especially depression is rare in third world countries including India. There are many studies including a number of Indian ones on the symptomatology of affective disorders especially depression from India. However, there has been considerable degree of confusion with respect to the depressive illness because of the differing conceptual approaches and terminologies used by different psychiatrists. Whatever the terminology used, a major depressive episode has got certain core symptoms like depressed mood, loss of interest and self esteem and certain biological symptoms like sleep disturbances and poor appetite.

Some of the characteristics of depression in our culture, in comparison with western culture, are (a) tendency for increased somatisation, (b) preponderance of paranoid ideas, (c) rarity of guilt feeling, and (d) low suicide rate. It is not uncommon in our culture to find depressives presenting with somatic complaints alone. Usual somatic complaints include vague and persistent aches and pains, tiredness, sleeplessness, poor appetite, poor sexual desire and constipation. Preponderance of these somatic symptoms make them seek consultation of general practitioners. It has been established that many of the chronic patients of general practitioners suffer from primary depressive disorder manifesting with somatic complaints. In many such cases it will be possible to elicit psychological symptoms of depression like depressed mood, worthlessness; hopelessness and at times even suicidal ideas on direct probing. However, in a few cases somatic symptoms are the only manifestation of depression so as to warrant a label of masked depression'. Persistent pain syndromes are the most common form of presentations of masked depression. Typical is the case of a 45-year-old man who suffered from 'atypical trigeminal neuralgia' and did not respond to usual treatment but showed complete recovery with antidepressants.

Persecutory ideations and delusions sometimes associated with hallucinations are reported to occur more frequently in our country. The distinction of such cases from schizophrenia and other paranoid psychosis is possible based on the contents of the hallucinations and delusions as well as patient's reaction to it. The voices are usually described to be derogatory and accusatory and on the whole congruent with the depressed mood. It can also be observed that with the clearing of depression all these hallucinations and delusions disappear completely.

It has been customary among sociologists and social psychiatrists to distinguish between 'guilt-culture' under which category were included the western and predominantly Christian cultures and 'shame cultures' which denoted the oriental cultures like Indian and Chinese. Western depressives have more feelings of guilt and remorse having sinned against God than depressives in the eastern countries. This has been attributed to the stress on personal responsibility, concept of original sin, etc. in the western countries. On the other hand, eastern societies tend to underplay the individual's responsibility and his actions and the society is more collective. This attitude tends to generate less guilt, and guilt and sin are not often expressed by depressives in our country. Many patients attribute their sufferings as punishments meted out for accumulated sins of previous births.

Depression accounts for the bulk of completed suicides in western countries, where the suicide rate in affective disorders is around 10–15%. On the other hand, Indian studies report very low suicide rates. It is our observation that though suicidal ideas are frequent, patients are prevented from active suicidal behaviour by a variety of factors, the so called 'suicide counters' described by Venkoba Rao. These include moral and spiritual attitude and factors of children, family, etc.

Manic episodes being more endogenously determined have got more or less similar characteristics in all cultures like cheerfulness, hyperactivity and grandiosity. There may also be fleeting delusions or hallucinations. Again the contents of the above symptoms will be congruent with the prevailing. mood of euphoria and are consistent with its social and cultural background. For example, it is common to find an Indian villager who claims to be possessed by his or her local diety and who claims to communicate with it and of possessing supernatural powers.

## NEUROTIC AND SOMATOFORM DISORDERS

The common disorders traditionally described are: (1) Phobic and other anxiety disorder, (2) Dissociative disorder, (3) Obsessive compulsive disorder, (4) Somatoform disorder. All these are met within our society. Culture modifies the symptoms in these also.

Anxiety disorder presents with pervasive feeling of anxiety, inability to relax and anxious expectation. These are accompanied with somatic symptoms like headache and other tension, pains, palpitation, tremulousness, excessive sweating, and other hyperadrenergic manifestations. It is quite common for the patients to elaborate these somatic accompaniments which are more concrete. Many patients especially illiterate will have difficulty in elaborating the more subtle and abstract physiological feelings of anxiety. The concepts of traditional Indian medicine also influence the way of expressing symptoms. This is especially common in hypochondriacal patients who usually refer these to the various vagaries of the humours—'Vatha', 'Pitha', and 'Kapha', in their bodies.

It is well established that the nature of hysterical symptoms is related to the patient's cultural, intellectual and social backgrounds. The more primitive the culture, the cruder the symptoms usually are. Thus many of the 'classical' hysterical symptoms like convulsions, paralysis, astasia-abasia-ataxia, blindness, etc. have become increasingly rare in western countries but are quite common still in our countries. Hysterical fainting and other dissociation states are also quite common. It is needless to say that these patients first go to a general practitioner or depending on the nature of disability to one or more specialists. It is usual for many patients to have undergone many protracted investigations before an organic condition is excluded and psychiatric referral made.

Much time and energy of both the physicians can be saved if the emotional settings in which many of these symptoms occur are gone into and a psychiatric diagnosis made based on these positive evidence than the usual practice of exclusion of all possible organic conditions.

Obsessive compulsive disorder is usually a chronic condition characterised by obsessions, compulsion or both. Obsessions are recurrent ideas or images which are irrelevant and irrational and occur against patient's conscious resistance. Compulsions are irresistible inner urges to perform certain acts often in a ritualistic way. The themes of these are taken from the culture. For example, an orthodox Hindu Brahmin was so much obsessed with the idea of cleanliness and doubts about pollution by untouchables that he had to spend most part of his day in repeated bathings.

Addictions. Some of the addictive agents like alcohol, cannabis, and opium have been in use in our country for centuries. Drugs like amphetamines, tranquillizers, and pethidine injection of morphine, mandrax, etc. are relatively new entrants into the field. Addictions to all these agents are found almost exclusively among males in our country.

Alcoholism is frequent equally in the rural and urban population. The usual presentations of alcoholism are alcoholic deterioration resulting in economic, occupational and social disruptions and withdrawal states with symptoms like tremulousness or 'shakes', insomnia, and restlessness. Delirium tremens is not that rare and a serious withdrawal symptom. Alcoholic hallucinosis is a condition resembling schizophrenic illness and is characterised by hallucinations mainly auditory. This condition can occur either during a withdrawal phase or during a drinking bout. Chronic alcoholism also can lead to a state of morbid sexual jealousy characterised by violent delusions of marital infidelity (Othello syndrome). A few alcoholics show an interesting pattern in their drinking habit. Periods of excessive and uncontrollable drinking alternate with long periods of abstinence in them. This dipso-manic pattern is believed to be a depressive equivalent and responds well to anti-depressants. Cannabis abuse, mainly ganja smoking, is quite frequent among students. Cannabis gives rise to transient psychotic state in some. Drugs like amphetamines, tranqui-llizers, Methaqualone have also become an 'in-thing' among students. Certain occupations add to the vulnerability, for example, hospital staff to pethidine and morphine, and bootleggers and bartenders to alcohol. Psychedelic drugs like LSD and mescaline are used only by a select band in our community.

### Suicidal Behaviour

Suicidal behaviour in India is essentially an adolescent phenomenon unlike in western countries where the aged population form the vulnerable group. As already mentioned depressives form only a small percentage of attempted and "complete suicide" in India unlike in western countries.

Certain cultural factors like family ties, moral beliefs, etc. play a role in preventing many suicides: It is also observed that many of the suicidal attempts among adolescents and young adults have an 'appeal' character rather than real intention to die. This appeal or 'cry for help' is usually directed towards one of the 'key' people in the family. The above discussion is not meant to underplay the seriousness of suicidal risk in any group of psychiatric patients and the risk of each case has to be assessed on individual merit.

### Culture-bound Syndromes

Certain syndromes, though basically belonging to one of the usual categories of psychiatric disorders, bear such a heavy stamp of a particular culture that they are called culture-bound syndromes. They are specific syndromes restricted to the setting of that particular culture. Many such exotic syndromes are described. They include 'Koro', a panicky state with fear of one's penis shrinking into the abdomen found in ethnic Chinese in Malaya. 'Latah', a form of startle reaction in Malayasia, 'Windigo' or morbid fear of cannibalism in certain Amerindian tribes, 'Piblokto' (Arctic-hysteria), a dissociative state found in 'Eskimos'. Possession states, 'Dhat syndrome' and 'Suchi-bai', are the common culture bound syndromes described in our country. Among these, possession states are the most frequently met with and are common in many of the other developing countries in Asia and Africa. 'Possession' basically is a dissociated state in which the subject is in a state of 'trance'. He or she often identifies with, or acts as a via medium with certain Gods, Goddesses, spirits or ancestors. Usually a part of hysterical disorder, possession can occur in schizophrenics, manics, and sometimes even in epileptics. 'Komarams' or 'Velichapads' in our society are professionals with a capacity to enter into a trance state and be possessed.

'Dhat' syndrome denotes the morbid fear of loss of vital energy in the form of semen usually by nocturnal emission or masturbation. Many of these patients complain of lethargy, lack of energy and will have a plethora of fears about bodily disability including fear of impotence, and fear of insanity. Symptoms of anxiety will be evident and guilt over masturbation can be elicited in many. 'Suchi-bai' is a morbid preoccupation with cleanliness described in Bengalis, but an equivalent form, colloquially referred to as 'Jalapisachu' is observable in higher castes of our society.

Majority of our population still do not consider mental illness as a disease at par with bodily diseases. Magico-religious theories like effect of black magic, possession by spirits, or punishments meted out for violation of taboos, etc. are still adhered to by many as explanations for cases where there are gross behavioural changes along with theories rooted on the humoural concepts, those of 'Vatha', 'Pitha', and 'Kapha'. On the other hand, where there are physical symptoms to the forefront as in hysteria and anxiety neurosis. The tendency is to attribute these somatic symptoms to some underlying physical ailments.

Culture bound syndromes are heterogeneous in their aetiology and presentation. However, they share some common features.

1. The affected patients are generally young.

2. They present with prominent somatic symptoms.

3. The symptoms invariably attract cultural attention.

4. There are no psychotic symptoms.

5. The condition does not lead to personality deterioration.

6. Aetiology often point to cultural attributes.

Culture is the sum total of the way of living of a group of people and psychiatric disorders are only one aspect, though morbid, of the way of living. In this frame of reference the symptoms become more meaningful and help to formulate the management strategies more effectively.

## FURTHER READING

1. Neppe, Tucker. Atypical unusual and cultural psychosis. In: Harold Kaplan, Benjamin Sadock eds, Comprehensive textbook of psychiatry. 5th ed, Vol.1,1989.

# 16

# Psychological Assessments in the Clinic

K P Abdul Salam

Psychological assessment of a person begins from the moment he enters the clinic and continues till he leaves the consulting room. This most usually consists of drawing inferences regarding the person's behaviour from what is observed in the consultation room. Structured psychological assessments are available today to assess the level of intellectual functioning, assess for learning disabilities, to assess and rate motivation for treatment, to help the clinician reach a formal diagnosis and so on. However, this chapter doesn't deal with such structured assessments. The kinds of assessments dealt with here are the ones which could help the clinician reach some form of initial hypothesis from clinical observations and case history without the use of formal testing.

## Adult Mental Retardation

As mentioned, there are various tests available to formally rate the level of intellectual functioning of a person and yield a definite IQ score. However, it is possible to reach a crude conclusion regarding the level of mental retardation from simple clinical observations and case history. Since IQ level can vary much with age, only adult mental retardation is taken into consideration here.

## Mild Mental Retardation

This is the old category of 'educable' persons. This suggests that they could be trained and educated with the help of 'special' training to compensate for their difficulties. As for the

245

developmental history, they are usually described as 'slow' in all activities. Many a times, these are perceived by caretakers as being 'lazy' and are not understood as real deficits. Patients with mild mental retardation are usually adept at independent self care and practical skills, but have difficulties where abstract thinking is involved. This is most usually evident in situations involving mental operations such as calculations. Therefore, he/she might be good at washing own clothes, but is unable to calculate balance during shopping or do the calculations required in tailoring. A usual experience reported in cooking is where the person is capable of following another adult's instructions properly but is unable to judge the right amount of salt and other ingredients to be added. During the interview, they might be able to give their address or write their name but are unable to do mental calculations. They might be able to perform well during initial school years but their performance decreases over time. Usually, parents report that they were good in academic performance nursery classes and first grade, but started to deteriorate from second grade.

## Moderate Mental Retardation

This is the 'trainable' category in the educational classification. These persons can be trained some simple skills, but are usually unable to complete formal academic education. Dysmorphic features could be seen in such individuals. Self care is never completely achieved and some might need supervision throughout life. Generally, they are able to move around in their neighbourhood, is able to engage in pre-adolescent play and is able to communicate their needs. During the interview, the individual might be able to answer simple questions such as giving their name or where they come from; but usually are unable to engage in a meaningful conversation. Many of these individuals are able to respond in monosyllables. However, he/she might need assistance in bathing, brushing and other motor activities. They are usually unable to do complex calculations, make purchases or grasp the concept of time.

## Severe Mental Retardation

This is the category of 'dependant'. These individuals usually have a history of delay in speech and motor milestones. Parents usually perceive a difference between this individual and other children of similar age from childhood itself. Usually, they are unable to carry out activities of daily living on their own. Therefore, they need assistance in activities such as brushing, bathing and eating. They are usually unable to help themselves at meals, unable to use simple tools such as knife, use pen/pencil for writing and go about the neighbourhood on their own.

## Profound Mental Retardation

These individuals often need assistance in all walks of life. There is usually a history of marked delay in developmental milestones. They might have difficulties in climbing the stairs, dressing oneself up, in washing own hands or talk in simple sentences. During the interview, it might be difficult to engage them in any form of communication. These individuals require structured routine and environment so that their needs could be taken care of. They are mostly placed in rehabilitation and day care settings to achieve this.

## Motivation

Clinically, motivation is understood as the extent to which a person desires change. In mental health field, motivation to change one's behavior is discussed the most in substance dependence syndromes. As is obvious, it is expected that any form of intervention is likely to effective only as much as the client is motivated. Resistance to treatment has been discussed in psychiatry since the inception of psychoanalytic ideas. During those times, it was seen to emerge from some unconscious forces. It was considered the duty of the therapist to unravel these unconscious motives behind resistance and help the client sustain motivation to change oneself. Recent models have, however, tried to put greater emphasis on the personal responsibility of the person in bringing about change.

## Transtheoretical Model

A popular model used in assessing and understanding motivation is Prochaska and DiClement's (1983) 'Stages of change' model. This model understands motivation as a dynamic state and the person is thought to be move between various stages of change. This is thought to be an improvement over viewing motivation in dichotomous categories of 'motivated' or 'unmotivated'. The transtheoretical model identifies five stages of change:

## 1. Precontemplation

This is the stage where the person has not considered any change. The client hardly acknowledges that substance use is a problem and is not bothered by it. Therefore, during the clinical interview, the patient would exhibit an attitude of carelessness towards the issue. When asked, 'what brought you here?' They might respond with issues other than the substance *per se*. They might point out other issues like marital conflicts or lack of appetite but not the substance use. Some of these patients might omit informing the clinician about the use of the substance. Only with specific questions might they give information regarding this. Some might have been brought forcefully by their relatives or have come only since their physician referred them. Some might just respond with 'I don't know'. There could be others who would agree with the clinician that the substance use is a problem, just for the sake of it. All of these are clues suggesting that the patient is in a Precontemplation stage. At this stage, the clinician is supposed to educate the patient regarding the harmful effects of being dependent on the substance.

## 2. Contemplation

This is the second stage of change where the patient has started considering change. The person has started thinking about the issue and has started to acknowledge it as a problem. The patient has engaged in a "pros-cons" analysis and has taken the costs and benefits of changing the behavior into account. At this stage, the client might readily agree that the substance use is a problem but might not be very sure about the steps to be taken towards changing it. Patients could respond with helplessness or overconfidence. Both could be an indication of having poorly considered concrete steps to change. Attributing one's substance to external situations such as family conflicts or giving overgeneralized statements such as 'I have the ability to stop using it whenever I want' are indications of poor motivation. When asked about the steps taken to reduce the dependence, concrete answers are rare. For most of them at this stage, change still is an abstract idea.

## 3. Determination

Determination is the third stage where the patient has thought about change in a concrete manner. The person considered the costs and benefits of the substance use and has decided to quit. The person starts making concrete plans of bringing about changes. This could include plans to bring about changes in one's lifestyle, social circles, family life, daily routine and so on. Usually, the person understands that change is a complex phenomenon and is ready to do 'all that it takes'. During the interview, the person might admit the substance dependence as a problem and would be able to tell the clinician about the changes he considers bringing about. Some of the patients at this stage might be frank enough to seek the clinician's help and suggestions in chalking out changes in his/her behavior.

## 4. Action

This is the stage where all the previous efforts come to fruition. The patient actually makes changes in his/her behaviour. Usually, there is a change in the general outlook of the patient towards various aspects of life. There could be changes in the financial, social, family and other areas. The patient would be in a position to tell the clinician about the concrete changes that he/she had made towards reducing dependence. The attitude exhibited is most often that of cautious optimism. The person is optimistic about stopping the substance use but not so hopeful that it is unrealistic. Patients at this stage accept their personal responsibility in bringing about change and usually do not exhibit overconfidence in doing so.

## 5. Maintenance

During the maintenance phase, the person continues the healthy lifestyle and maintains abstinence. The person typically has found the alternate lifestyle better and fulfilling. He/she may start involving himself/herself in 'positive addictions' and engage in community activities. Usually the improvement is corroborated by the relatives and significant other.

## Specific Learning Disabilities

Specific learning disabilities (SLD) represent difficulties in acquisition of scholastic skills such as reading, spelling and arithmetic. ICD-10 specifies that the severity of skill-deficits should be clinically significant in the absence of mental retardation and physical causes such as visual or hearing impairments. The deficit shouldn't be a direct cause of lack of learning opportunities or training. In our country, there are a few tests available to formally assess and rate SLD. Clinician's judgements and assessments can provide valuable additional data.

One of the most important points to check for is whether the difficulties are present from early school days. If a student was able to perform well till 8th grade, but has poor performance since then, it is most likely due to factors (such as lack of tuitions or practice) than due to learning disabilities.

Clinically, the student can be asked to read some paragraphs from his/her book, do simple written calculations and write some words to dictation. If the client performs too far below the expected performance for his/her grade, a learning disability should be suspected. A rule of thumb is to check whether the person is able to perform at least two grades below the current level. If not, SLD could be thought of. The clinician should, therefore, have some working knowledge regarding the school curriculum.

As for reading, some clues are important. Lack of fluency in reading, reading word by word, spelling out the words, guessing words or omitting some of the words are indications of a learning disability. An extremely important deficit seen is the inability to use phonetic cues to read. Most of us are able to read new words using the phonetic cues available in the word. In languages like Malayalam or Tamil, this is evident as difficulties in grasping the idea of *dheergam* or students with learning disability might not be able to do so. Importantly, students with learning disability might display a poor comprehension of what they have read. It seems that in their struggle to connect words to read, they lose the meaning of what they have read. Clinically, when asked about the meaning of what they just read, most of the clients would want to read the material a second or third time to decipher the meaning.

In spelling, students with learning disability have similar difficulties. However, they are usually good at using phonetic cues. Specific learning disability in reading should be ruled out before diagnosing a person as having SLD in spelling. SLD in reading itself is known to be associated with spelling errors. However, these tend to be phonetically inaccurate. Clinically, when there are difficulties such as missing out a letter, adding or substituting a letter, missing punctuations and wrong capitals, an independent SLD in spelling should be considered. Clients with SLD in spelling also might have difficulty in expressing their ideas using meaningfully structured sentences.

Students with SLD in arithmetic might show difficulties in the basic mathematical operations such as additions and subtractions. In the current system, it is expected that a student gains the required skills to perform graded multiplications at least by the sixth grade. When the student is unable to perform so, SLD should be considered. However, the clinician should keep in mind that the performance can vary based on the child's current grade and age and judge accordingly.

Thus, this chapter dealt with three important areas of clinical assessment carried out by practitioners on a daily basis. As mentioned, the aim was not to discuss the use of formal testing and objective scales to assess these aspects. The idea was to discuss how these aspects could be assessed in a clinical interview. These assessments provide rich information and help the clinician to form some initial hypothesis regarding the patient's state. They provide information which could enhance the date obtained through formal assessments and thus can help in formulating a treatment plan.

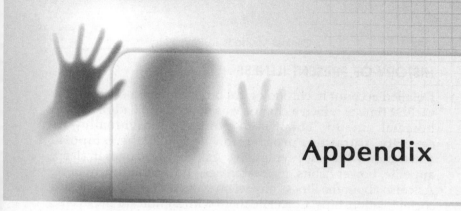

# Appendix

# SEVANA HOSPITAL AND RESEARCH CENTRE

PATTAMBI

## DEPARTMENT OF MENTAL HEALTH

HOSP. NO. _____ COMPUTER CODE _____ DATE _____

NAME _____ SEX _____ AGE _____ DOB _____

FATHER'S NAME / MOTHER'S NAME _____

MARITAL STATUS: SINGLE / MARRIED / SEPARATED / DIVORCED / WIDOWED

RESIDENCE: RURAL / URBAN / SUB-URBAN SOCIOECONOMIC STATUS

_____

ADDRESS _____ name, relation to patient _____

_____ intimacy, impression of _____

_____ informant's reliability _____

_____  _____

PIN _____ REFERAL (source _____

PHONE _____ of and reasons for) _____

OCCUPATION _____

COMPLAINTS (Symptoms in chronological order with duration and mode of onset (acute, gradual, insidious) of each. Complaints volunteered by the patient and revealed by questioning should be recorded separately preferably in their own words).

**PRECIPITATING FACTORS**

# HISTORY OF PRESENT ILLNESS

Detailed account in chronological order of the illness from the earliest time at which a change was noticed until admission to hospital. Enquire about each symptom individually—its severity, duration, progression and also the temporal association with other symptoms. Ask about changes in sleep, appetite, bowel habits, interest in sex and sexual functioning. Ask also about the illness impact on patient's family, work and social relationships. Correlate them with significant life events like death, financial setbacks, shifting of residence, change of jobs, concurrent illness, etc. Enquire about any treatment taken and its effect on the symptoms.

# FAMILY HISTORY

### PARENTS

Consanguinity. Age or age at the time of death with cause of death. Health, occupation, personality, separation from the parents. Parent's relationship with one another. Separations, divorce or remarriage.

### SIBS

In chronological order with names, ages, marital status, occupation, personality and health. Patient's relationship with siblings—well adjusted/sibling rivalry?

### HOME ATMOSPHERE

Salient happenings in family during patient's early years. Family beliefs, eccentricities. Race and religion. Social position of family.

### FAMILY HISTORY OF PSYCHIATRIC AND OTHER MEDICAL DISORDERS

Psychiatric disorder, personality disorder, epilepsy, alcoholism, drug dependence, suicide, mental retardation. Absconding from home? Neurological or medical disorders.

# PERSONAL HISTORY

## EARLY DEVELOPMENT

Details of pregnancy (planned or not) and birth. Habit training difficulties. Milestones (walking, talking, sphincter control, etc.) Precocious or retarded. Delicate or healthy as baby.

## HEALTH DURING CHILDHOOD

Infections, movement disorders, seizures. Hospitalisations. Effect of illness on development.

## CHILDHOOD NEUROTIC SYMPTOMS

Nocturnal enuresis, nightmares, thumb-sucking, nail-biting, sleepwalking, stammering, food fads, mannerisms and tantrums.

# EDUCATIONAL AND WORK HISTORY

## EDUCATION

Ages on starting and finishing, types of school, academic record, games and sports. Relationships with teachers and peers. Hobbies and interests. Nicknames, special abilities and disabilities. Failures.

## OCCUPATIONS

Chronological list of jobs held with reasons for change. Present financial circumstances. Satisfaction in job: Reasons for dissatisfaction. Ambitions.

# SEXUAL HISTORY

## MENSTRUAL HISTORY

Age at menarche. Regularity. Dysmenorrhea. Pre-menstrual tension. Age of menopause, menopausal symptoms.

## SEXUAL PRACTICES

Attitude towards sex. Adolescent and current sexual functioning. Masturbation. Guilt feelings? Homosexuality. Heterosexual experiences apart from marriage. Sexual fantasies. Perversions?

## MARITAL HISTORY

Age at marriage. How long known before marriage? Arranged marriage/love marriage? Forced by pregnancy? Present age, occupation, health and personality of spouse. Frequency and satisfaction of intercourse. Contraceptive measures. Children— ages, names, personality, health. Abortion. Patient's attitudes to children.

## PREVIOUS MEDICAL HISTORY

Illness, operations, accidents—dates, duration and hospitalization.

## PREVIOUS PSYCHIATRIC HISTORY

Nature and duration of illness, date, duration and nature of any treatment. Outcome. Details of all psychiatric symptoms for which treatment was not given (insomnia, mood variations, obsessional and anxiety symptoms, etc.)

## PREMORBID PERSONALITY
### (Give descriptive examples)

**Social:** Friends : Few or many? superficial or close? own sex or opposite sex? work and workmates; clubs, societies.

**Use of leisure:** Hobbies or interests.

**Mood:** Cheerful, despondent, anxious, worrying, irritable, optimistic, pessimistic, self-depreciative, satisfied, over-confident, stable, fluctuant (with or without any reason) controlled, demonstrative.

**Character:** Timid reserved, shy, self-conscious, sensitive; suspicious, jealous, resentful, quarrelsome, irritable, impulsive, selfish; dependent, strict, fussy, rigid; meticulous, punctual, excessively tidy.

**Habits:** Food, excretory functions, alcohol, tobacco, sleep, self-medication.

**Energy:** Initiative, energetic or sluggish, fatigability

**Fantasy:** Extent, content.

**Attitudes and standards:** Moral and religious

# EXAMINATION OF MENTAL STATE

## APPEARANCE, BEHAVIOUR

Description as complete and life-like as possible of what is observed in patient's appearance and behaviour. Particulars of body build, posture, clothes and grooming, facial appearance. Psychomotor behaviour, gait, level of activity, movements. Interpersonal behaviour and attitude towards examiner. Level of rapport and eye contact.

## COGNITIVE STATUS

**Sensorium:** Comatose/stuporois/drowsy/alert

**Attention and concentration attention:** Easily aroused and sustained/distractible/pre-occupied. simple tests: Digit span test, serial subtraction test (e.g. serial seven test), spelling words backwards, reciting the days of the week/months of the year in reverse order. Both accuracy and speed of performance are observed.

**Orientation:** Patient's awareness of person, place, time and social context. Self/person/place/time/day/date/month/year/social context. If unable to answer these correctly, ask about his/her own identity.

**Memory:** Immediate/recent/remote. Effect of deficit on patient. Attitude towards deficit. Simple tests: name and address repeated immediately and after five minutes. Three words recalled after three minutes. Sequences of digits forwards and backwards.

## GENERAL INFORMATION AND INTELLIGENCE

Questions should have some relevance to the patient's educational and cultural background. Note down patient's level of formal education and self education: Estimate of the patient's intellectual capacity (vocabulary, interpretation of proverbs, calculations): General knowledge.

## MOOD

Subjective: patient's own assessment of his/her mood.
Objective: Observed by the examiner. Note down the predominant mood (calm, depressed, irritable, anxious, fearful,

terrified, angry, happy, elated, euphoric, apathetic), changeability: monotonic/labile. Appropriateness; appropriate or inappropriate.

## PERCEPTION

**Sensory distortions:** Changes in intensity/quality/spatial/form.

## SENSORY DECEPTION

Illusions. Hallucinations.
Individual senses: Hearing, vision, smell, touch, taste. Pain, deep sensations, vestibular. Special kinds of hallucinations: Functional/reflex/extracampine/autoscopy. Find out the content and circumstances of occurrence. Patient's attitude towards and explanation about them.

## OTHER PERCEPTUAL EXPERIENCES:

Depersonalization, derealization, *deja vu*, *jamais vu*, micropsia, macropsia.

## PATIENT'S ATTITUDE TO PERCEPTUAL DISTURBANCES

### SPEECH

How the patient speaks is recorded under this heading, whereas what the patient says is recorded under disorders of thought.

**Reaction time:** Slow/quick. Spontaneity. Spontaneous/non-spontaneous/hesitant.

**Productivity:** Monosyllabic/elaborate/pressure of speech.

**Pitch:** Monotonous/whispered/loud. Speed: Fast/slow.

**Articulation**: Slurring/stammering/dysarthria.

Anything notable about vocabulary, choice of words. Record a sample of conversation/speech/talk for a detailed analysis.

### THOUGHT

From the quality of speech and writings the interviewer makes inferences about the process of thinking and cognitive organization. Stream: Flight of ideas/retardation/circumstantiality/thought blocking. Form: Poverty of thought/ poverty of content of thought/tangentiality/derailment/ incoherence/illogicality/clang associations/neologism/word approximation/echolalia/stilted speech/self reference/ paraphasia/stereotypy/perseveration/concreteness over inclusiveness.

**Possession—obsessions and compulsions:** "Do any thoughts keep coming into your mind, even though you try hard not to have them?" If the answer is "yes", ask for an example. "Do you have to do things over and over again when most people would have done them only once?" Give examples.

**Thought alienation:** Insertion, withdrawal, broadcasting.

**Preoccupations:** About the illness/environmental problems/depressive ideas/phobias/hypochondriacal ideas. Delusions. Persecution/love/jealousy/grandeur/ill health/ guilt/nihilism/poverty. Mood-congruent or incongruent Systematized delusions: Shared delusions

**Abstract thinking:** It is helpful to ask the patient the meaning of various proverbs and record his/her answers verbatim to assess the capacity for abstract thinking.

### INSIGHT AND JUDGEMENT

Degree of awareness and understanding the patient has that he/she is ill. Assess social and test judgements. Does the patient have reasonable plans for the future?

### COMMENTS AND DIAGNOSTIC FORMULATION

### PROVISIONAL DIAGNOSIS

### TARGET SYMPTOMS

### HISTORY TAKEN BY

### Date

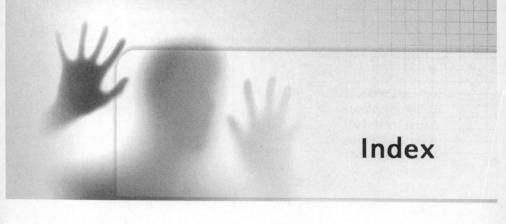

# Index

# B

# C

# V

# W